CRAFTING THE BODY DIVINE

RITUAL, MOVEMENT AND BODY ART

YASMINE GALENORN

THE CROSSING PRESS
FREEDOM, CALIFORNIA

Copyright © 2001 by Yasmine Galenorn
Cover and book design by Petra Serafim
Cover photo © Elyse Regehr/Stone
Interior illustrations by Petra Serafim
Author photo by Samwise Galenorn

Printed in the USA

For information on bulk purchases or group discounts for this and other Crossing Press
titles, please contact our Special Sales Director at 800/777-1048, Ext. 203.
www.crossingpress.com

Library of Congress Cataloging-in-Publication Data

Galenorn, Yasmine, 1961-
  Crafting the body divine : ritual, movement, and body art / by Yasmine Galenorn.
    p. cm.
  Includes bibliographical references and index.
  ISBN 1-58091-104-8 (pbk.)
  1. Magic. 2. Beauty, Personal--Miscellanea.   I. Title.
BF1623.B43 G35 2001
299--dc21

                                                                    2001047254

0   9   8   7   6   5   4   3   2   1

Acknowledgments

This book and its soon-to-be published companion, *Sexual Ecstasy and the Divine*, have not been easy to write. Aside from the obvious research needed, they were emotionally draining in many ways, even as they were exhilarating and fun. I give my deepest thanks to:

My husband, Samwise Galenorn, for everything—for support, for love, for telling me I'm beautiful and meaning it, even when I feel like a mess.

My interviewees: Ray, my tattooist, for whom I have the utmost respect and sincere gratitude for his willingness to be interviewed for this book; Sue, who has taught me more about strength through adversity than all the books in the world; "Shirley," a dear friend, whom I will always think of as a "secret jockette"; Kellie, my masseuse, who is helping me teach my body to relax; Youngtree, whom I learned from through friendship; and the numerous others who offered opinions, insight, and personal experiences to guide me through the labyrinth of the body divine.

I also wish to thank:

Kevin, my hairdresser, who has taught me the value of a good cut.

Offline and online friends, who offered emotional support during my writing and research:

Siduri, Lisa M., Johnny M., Daniela S., Thera P., Toby P., KG R., Ginger R., Saga D., Geoff D., Jenna, Red, Kate, Aaron E., Toni G., Robert L., Mark T., Nanette, Kelly A., Sorciere, Will R., Rehabber, Lori K., Craig K., and many more.

Thanks to all my readers who kept asking me when this book was coming out.

Many thanks to Astrid Sandell, for encouraging me to write on this subject.

As always, my deepest love I give to my Lord and Lady, Mielikki and Tapio, who live in my heart this twentieth year I've been in the Craft.

Dedicated to:
Shiva and Shakti
and all women and men who manifest the
face of the Goddess and the God
in their souls, hearts, and body.
This means *you*.

Contents

I am just a holy instrument of joy.

—*Shriekback: Go Bang*
"Big Fun"

Introduction

I hadn't thought of writing this book until one day, shortly before I got my third tattoo, the idea struck me like a thunderbolt from Big Daddy Zeus himself. I was meditating on my upcoming appointment with the needle, spending time in ritual welcoming the approaching energy, when it flashed through my mind how ancient an art this practice is. That led me to thinking about the body in ritual, which led me to thinking about dancing, body modification, beauty, and of course sex.

As Pagans, so much of our spirituality seems rooted in the world around us and yet we tend to focus on transcendence, on moving beyond our bodies even while we still profess a connection with the Earth at a physical level. I think perhaps this has come about in an attempt to divorce ourselves from superficialities. What we forget is that we are physical creatures for a reason: we are here in-body now.

It is easy for books like this to become judgmental: "If you don't do it my way, don't do it at all." This is one reason why I write my books based on personal experience. These are *my opinions,* from both my own life and from research I've done.

With *Crafting the Body Divine* and its sister book, *Sexual Ecstasy and the Divine,* I want to help you discover that we are each unique in body shape, color, size, and structure, and that we should take pride in the passion inherent in our bodies, no matter what we've been handed at birth. Fat, thin, tall, short, dark, light: we all belong to the human race and it's time we stopped letting these differences come between us.

Think how much freer we'd feel if we stopped loathing our bodies for not being like the latest supermodel or movie hunk. Think of the energy we could have if we celebrated our spirituality through our bodies and integrated the Divine spark of passion into our lives. Think of the understanding we could cultivate if we accept the differences of others and if our own were accepted in turn.

Please know that I cannot offer personal advice. I'm not a professional counselor, and I don't have the time, because of my writing and living my own life, to help others more than through the confines of this book and the information on my Web sites (see Galenorn En/Visions at http://www.galenorn.com for my various Web sites). If you wish to contact me about this or any of my books, you may do so care of the publishers, or through my e-mail: darkmoon@galenorn.com. If you wish to contact Ms. Alcorn (interviewed in chapter 3), you may e-mail her through me.

The body is more than just a vehicle for the soul—it is our home at this time. We must explore it, rejoice in it, and treat it with respect and passion, just as we do the primal energies of the God and Goddess—Fire and Water, yin and yang, polarities in conflict even as they embrace. Out of this embrace, we find creation. Bright Blessings and may your life be filled with joy.

Part I

~

FROM THE INSIDE OUT

The rose looks fair, but fairer we it deem
For that sweet odour which doth in it live.

—William Shakespeare, *Sonnet 54*

CHAPTER ONE

The Mirror of Beauty

Whilst burning through the inmost veil of heaven,
the soul of Adonis like a star
Beacons from the abode where the eternal are.
                              —Shelley, "The End of Adonis"

While many books focus on the history and politics of beauty, I think we need here an examination of attitude: a look at how we relate to society when it comes to beauty.

Most Americans tend to ignore the fact that our standards of beauty are not necessarily held worldwide. What we value is not always prized in other countries, and not everyone in the United States holds the stereotypical views on beauty, sexuality, and passion.

When you look at the standards of acceptability in other countries, especially non-Western nations, you begin to see that every kind of body, at one time or another, in one place or another, has been considered desirable. On a personal note, I've dated enough foreign men, as well as American men, to know this for a fact. Women who've visited Hawaii, Polynesia, Italy, and the Middle East have had to fight men off, even though the women are not what our society promotes as beautiful. My own husband doesn't know or care what the supermodels look like and has finally convinced me after years of being together that he really isn't interested in stick-figure women. He simply wants me to be happy, to feel and act like the sexy and strong woman I am.

Ten years ago, tattooed women were considered biker sluts and tattooed men were Hell's Angels. Today, tattoos have become the basis for an entire subculture and are going mainstream. The modern movement toward primitivism and tribalism has changed what is considered attractive. Boundaries are being broken, limitations challenged, and more women *and* men are refusing either to conform to the *Vogue* style of beauty or to be cast into the land of the undesirable. We seem to be making some change in the acceptance of other body types/colors/styles.

Of course, every generation will have a special look. There's not much we can do about it; there will always be fads and fashion trends. Some are fun to play with, some are ridiculous, a few are downright dangerous. But if we buck the trend, we can choose to take what works for us and leave the rest. When we develop a personal style that is truly comfortable and suits us, we never need to fear being out of touch with our inner selves. At the same time, we must be willing to experiment, to take a few risks, for we change as we grow and what was right for us ten years ago may not suit us now.

As we become comfortable with ourselves, as we project an aura of strength and self-confidence that is hard to shake, I believe we will see less condemnation of other people for the way they look and the lifestyles they lead. Within an environment where diversity rules, mutual tolerance and respect can flourish.

This is not to say that we will free ourselves of troublemakers. We can pretty much guarantee that there will always be malcontents, those whose insecurities and fears drive them to demean others constantly in order to shore up their own lackluster egos. We should simply accept the fact that this part of society has always been with us, is with us now, and will always be with us.

However, we do not have to accept their words as gospel, to turn their rage inward on ourselves. We need only accept what is true to our hearts, and the rest of society be hanged. Because, dear friends, when you really look at it, who will be your judge when you die? And when you leave this world, don't you want to have loved yourself and embraced life with a passion, rather than hiding shamefaced in your room?

There has been a strong movement in our spiritual circles to deny the importance of the body. I understand this to a degree. Partly this is an attempt to counter our tendency to conform to the current standard in our looks, our sexuality, and our body decoration. However, this philosophy leads to the denial of our physicality. This I find unacceptable. "Looks don't matter, it is what's inside that counts" is perhaps the most abused excuse we use to avoid connecting with our physical selves. This thought is a convenient way to avoid facing the reality that for the duration of our lives on this plane, we are corporeal beings and we are here to experience our connection to the world around us.

What people seem to ignore is that by changing our views about bodies, by getting to know them and reveling in them, we can overcome the stigma attached to being outside the norm. And while I am a staunch feminist, I think that in our attempts to equalize the situation between the sexes, we women have perhaps given away too much of our connection with our feminine and sexual selves.

An interesting note: recently (as of this writing), NOW (the National Organization for Women) has agreed to sanction the BDSM (bondage/domination/sadomasochism) movement as acceptable between men and women. For a while, they approved it as appropriate behavior for lesbians, but it was still considered a power and repression issue between men and women. Finally, NOW has realized that thousands of women choose this form of sexuality—they are not coerced into it. It is simply one of the myriad expressions of human passion.

GETTING IN TOUCH WITH YOURSELF

Before you can be fully comfortable with your sexuality and your body, you must be comfortable with yourself. This exercise is valuable for helping you get in touch with and make peace with your inner sense of being. I do this on a regular basis, at least a couple times a year, to ascertain whether or not my focus has changed and to reacquaint myself with who I really am.

You will need only yourself and a comfortable chair. Sit back, relax, and close your eyes. Visualize an office. Make it comfortable, with furniture that you like and a view through the window that speaks to your heart. See a large desk in the room, and behind the desk, a comfortable chair. Walk over to the chair and sit down.

The door opens and you see yourself walk in. Examine how you feel when you see yourself. Do you automatically pass a negative judgment? Do you wince? Are you seeing yourself as you truly are, or as you wish you would be? Try to see yourself in an honest, detached, non-judgmental way. You wouldn't automatically make snide remarks about a stranger, would you? And you wouldn't turn around and make a hurtful comment to a friend, would you? Vow to treat yourself at least as well as you would treat a friend.

Next, say hello to yourself, and begin asking some questions. Listen carefully, and don't try to respond with answers you think you should hear. Allow your subconscious to answer instead. Sometimes inner dreams, hopes, and desires are drowned in the flood of "shoulds." When we start telling ourselves we should be this and we should do that because society, friends, or family pressure us, we run the risk of losing touch with who we are.

You might ask some of the following questions:

- What do I want to do with the next year of my life?
- If I could travel to any place in the world, where would I go and why?
- Am I happy in my job? Why or why not? If not, what would I change so that I could be happy?
- Do I enjoy the friends I have made? Do I feel the need to expand my horizons—to meet new people? What kind of people do I want to pass my time with? Where might I meet them?
- If I am in a relationship, how do I feel about it? Am I comfortable or do I feel that something is lacking? Have my partner or I changed so much that we no longer connect? What can I do to get back on track?
- What about my spare time? Am I pursuing hobbies that I enjoy, or have I outgrown them? Is it time to learn something new?

Use these and other questions you come up with to see where you are now, if you are happy or if you are in a rut. Then sit down with a pen and paper and figure out what you can do to make your life flow in the direction you want it to flow. What changes can you make now? What changes will take time to implement? Are there aspects to your life that will require major thought and reconstruction? Use this exercise to help you delve into your subconscious, to discover what you really want now.

THE PC REVOLUTION

When I am honest with myself, I realize how tired I am of the PC revolution. No, not personal computers. Political correctness has at times become a method of harassing other people. There are some values that go far beyond the term. It is a moral choice to fight racism, sexism, hate crimes, or harassment because of disabilities.

I want to talk about the more subtle PCness. Bluntly put, I am not a man, nor do I wish to be treated like a man. Let me state up front, if I say "leave me alone" to some jerk and he doesn't, I'm going to stomp him. But I am so tired of seeing the men I meet tiptoe around because they're afraid I'm going to scream at them for holding a door open for me, for complimenting me, for winking at me.

And I'm equally irritated with the women who stare at me in disapproval when I wear a low-cut blouse or a long billowing skirt. I *like* being a woman, and I like being acknowledged as a woman. I love cosmetics, I revel in expensive perfume, I thrive on bantering and flirting. All are wonderful and fun if not abused. None of this lessens the fact that I'm a strong-willed and intelligent human being.

What has happened to our generation? We hype sex continuously in the magazines and media, yet avoid expressing our sexual selves in real life. We scream, "No, you can't say that," when a colleague tells us we look nice, yet we spend millions on products designed to make us more beautiful. The system is screwed up. We have to get our act together and find a healthier way to express ourselves. We must cut out the hypocrisy.

I once had a coworker who would occasionally whistle at me. Appropriate for the office? Maybe not. But I was never offended because he was nice and appreciative of the work that I did. He simply thought I was beautiful, and let me know. If I had told him to stop, he would have. He was that type of man. Today, I could have him fired for his behavior. But I wouldn't.

There is nothing wrong with someone acknowledging beauty. When will we get out of the rut we are in? How many women look like Cindy Crawford? How many men have abs of steel and square jaws? And frankly, who wants everyone to look like that anyway?

Don't you ever get tired of hearing women worry about being fat or having bad hair? Do you hear yourself lapse into the same rhetoric about your own body? And men are not immune to this, especially in today's world. They often feel too short, too bald, too pudgy, or too poor, or that their cocks are too small.

I know it's difficult, but to break free of the self-deprecating cycle and at the same time free others from judging you, you have to learn how to accept your state of being, make the most you can of what you have, and enjoy your body.

Let me put it this way: I am a fat, short, tattooed, long-haired, wickedly sensual, and highly intelligent Witch. And yet I am one of the most grounded people I know. Period. And none of those words, or the concepts behind them, contradict any of the others.

Face it…you have large breasts? They're probably not going to be perky unless you invest in silicone. You have hips? Well, hips mean thick thighs. You're a short man? That doesn't necessarily mean you're short in all areas, and believe me, size matters only when there's way too little or way too much. Quality, friends, that's what counts. Your attitude and the passion in your soul and heart will come through your body if you learn to give it free rein and expression. And it doesn't mean you have to act sleazy. It simply means that you can revel in your own passionate being in all areas of your life and let your energy flow without censoring yourself.

I want to see people revel in their beauty, in their passion, in their sensuality without putting down others who are different and censuring themselves. When you begin to enjoy your own sensuality, you will find you aren't nearly so threatened by others who do the same. To accept this side of yourself, to get to know your body, you manifest a self-empowerment that is hard for others to shake. You will feel less at the mercy of others' opinions when you begin to express your true and full nature.

For some, this will mean a natural, athletic look and attitude. For others, it will be a lush, opulent aura. Find what works for you, and ignore anyone who tells you that you aren't beautiful, sensual, or passionate. So damn it, haul out the perfume and the silk scarves, or the hiking boots and the sleeping bag, and enjoy your body! I hope that this book will help you discover your beauty and passion, and help you embrace it without shame.

Find your dance, and may it be ecstatic.

CHANGING PERSPECTIVE

"This is all fine and good," I can hear you saying. "It makes sense, yes, but how do I get the attitude and keep it?" I'm not going to lie and say that with one of my rituals—wham, bam, you'll be in heaven, ma'am. The kind of attitude that makes people stand up and take notice, the kind of attitude that lasts, requires time and perseverance, but is worth the effort. Pray tell me what use is it to go through life uncertain and unhappy with yourself? It takes just as much energy to continue being depressed as it does to work your way out of that cellar.

Yes, you will have to work to develop an attitude which sparks interest and respect, but, remember, if you allow yourself to remain mired in depression and low self-esteem, you'll feel eaten from the inside out. This drain of energy affects every part of your life and interferes with your work, your social life, your spiritual growth, and your general sense of well-being. Attitude has also been linked to health; those with a better outlook on life tend to heal faster from injuries and illnesses.

When you walk into a room, when you speak, when you write a letter, even when you go into an online chat room, you want to be strong without overwhelming others. You need to stand apart, to find your unique style without coming on as obnoxious or pretentious. There's a certain feeling to this attitude, a smile on the inside that says, "I know I'm good and I'm not worried about whether others figure it out or not. The ones who do will be my friends, the ones who don't will go their own way at no loss to me."

Attitude starts on the inside, of course. Without that core, without that sense of self, even the most classically beautiful people lack fire and substance. They will pale and fade in the light of someone who, while perhaps not reflecting the mainstream of beauty/good looks, radiates and sustains power and passion.

To discover beauty within yourself, you must also discover it in others who do not fit the stereotypes. I have been cruising the Internet for almost two years. During that time, I've encountered hundreds of Web sites out there, and yes, some are sex sites. Others are more artistic, where the women and men pictured are not your typical *Playboy* types. Some of these sites charge money to join. If people pay to see women and men who are not Miss April and Mr. Olympia, then you know there are people out there who appreciate all body types.

I suggest that you start buying magazines that promote alternative lifestyles, alternative fashions, other body types than what the fashion slicks offer. I'm not saying you have to give up your *Marie Claire* or your *Penthouse*; just start familiarizing yourself with other body types so they won't seem so strange.

For those of us who do not fit the stereotypical image of beauty, it can be disconcerting to see images in print that are similar to our body types that are not being vilified or ridiculed. It takes time to get used to it, but eventually you will come to appreciate it. When I first saw *BBW Magazine,* I was stunned that these women could be so beautiful and yet still large. I felt the same about *Radiance Magazine.* Now, the large-sized women in *Mode* look like most of the normal women I see around me and I find the fashion slicks totally unrealistic. I seldom read them except for the articles on cosmetics and skin care.

When I started reading tattoo magazines, it took me a little while to adjust to seeing bodies as canvas for art. Some forms of body modification still don't work for me, still leave me wincing; I can't imagine myself going to certain lengths. However, I have a number of friends who are into extreme body modification. They approach the practice most often for spiritual reasons. This has led me to a point where I accept the brandings and scarifications while understanding that I do not have to adopt them into my own life. We must restructure our views of normality and what is acceptable. We must reach out to understand others on a deeper level before we can grasp their need for such unique personal expression.

Because my tattoos are large and quite prominent, when I walk into a store or down the street, I get looks from just about everyone I meet. I've seen everything from disgust, to fear, to lust, to appreciation. I've learned to dismiss those people who automatically turn away in distaste. I wouldn't want them in my life with that attitude.

This isn't to say you will be attracted to every body type, nor should you expect to be. People do have natural tendencies and turn-ons. There is no denying this. However, I think that we need to expand our vision of what we find attractive or merely acceptable. This also helps us when we confront cultural differences. If we transcend the fear of what is different, if we search for the beauty in our opposites, we expand our horizons and, in turn, lessen the tension in this world.

Visualization to Remove Prejudices

Relax and get comfortable. You need to use this exercise when you are feeling grounded. Visualize looking at yourself in a mirror. See yourself as you are. Try to remain detached, without any judgments about your body. Now imagine that you are changing color. If you are white, see yourself first as you might look if you were Asian. Then see yourself as if you were black. Wherever you start, I want you to visualize yourself as a different race and see how it would feel to be you. How do you think your friends would treat you? How would you treat others? Examine your feelings toward people of a different race or ethnicity.

Now, see yourself as you actually are. This time, visualize changing genders. How would you look as a man? As a woman? What do you think you would feel like? How do you react to people of the opposite gender? Do you demean them? Do you devalue them? Do you enjoy their company? How do you feel if someone puts you in a category as "woman" or "man"? Examine your feelings toward the opposite sex.

Once again, return to your normal state. Now see yourself changing shape. First see yourself as growing fatter. Try to appreciate the curves on your body. How does it feel to have more flesh? What are some of the benefits of being larger? Now think of how you react to people who are plump or fat. Do you laugh at them? Do you shy away? Do they attract you? Examine your feelings toward those who aren't thin.

Once more, return to your normal state. This time see yourself getting thinner. Feel the difference it would make to have less flesh on your body. Try to appreciate the benefits of this body type. Now think about how you react to people who are thin. Do you admire their bodies more than you admire others? Do you find them less appealing? Examine your attitudes toward those who are slender.

Finally, look into the mirror and see yourself as you are again. Now if you are able-bodied, find yourself sitting in a wheelchair. If you are disabled, find yourself standing strong. How does it feel to view the world through the eyes of someone who is different than you? What challenges do you face? How would your friends react to you? How do you react to others who are different than yourself? Do you find yourself getting impatient with their pace, or their attitudes toward the body and movement? Do you understand that this is simply another way of being human? Examine your feelings and potential prejudices against disability or mobility.

When you've finished this exercise, take a few moments to reevaluate how you react to those who are different than you. Often society tends to desexualize those people who are fat or disabled or old. This is a sad prejudice, leading to many heartaches and low self-esteem. If you share some of these automatic assumptions, what can you do to clear them out of your life? By allowing others to be fully human, happy, and sexual in their lives, no matter what their situation is, you also give yourself permission to be an integrated and happy individual.

LEARNING TO APPRECIATE YOUR BODY

Once you've started seeing your beauty in a wide variety of styles, looks, colors, and attitudes, you are on your way to appreciating yourself. The basic key to accepting yourself is this: you have to want to accept yourself. You have to decide to quit being a victim of society's whims. You have to work at it.

There is no simple way, no magic formula to make you love yourself overnight. I'm sorry, there isn't. However, you can achieve this state if you accept the fact that you'll have to work at it and shed tears over it. You'll backslide and have days when you look in the mirror and wince. Everyone does—you wouldn't be human if you didn't. But you can change your attitude about yourself if you make up your mind to start living now instead of waiting for the magical day when you will suddenly blossom and step into a new skin. Just like any goal in life, there may never be a someday. Start living now for the present, because you can never count on the future. Tomorrow you could die in a bus crash, tomorrow war could erupt, tomorrow the sun could fade, the dreamer awaken, and this beautiful, ecstatic vision we call life could expire and become one faded memory.

You have four good limbs, you can see to read this book, you have your mental faculties, you can hear? Well, damn it, what are you complaining about? You can't fit into a size four dress, let alone a size fourteen? Tough. You don't need a large-sized condom? Tough. You have a birthmark, you have freckles, hips, thighs, heavy breasts that sag a bit, you wear glasses? Deal with it. Live with being human and make the most out of your life. Find the beauty in your body. Curves are sexy. Birthmarks make you unique. Breasts that aren't perky are large and sensuous and so much fun to touch.

And what if you are in a wheelchair? Life sucks sometimes. It isn't fair, no it's not. But there are athletes who have missing limbs. They ski. They compete in marathons. They are in love, are loved, and have children. Accept where you are, and learn to overcome those boundaries which you can transcend.

Life is to be lived, to be experienced. Throw yourself in and feel the passion of the drumbeat that is the beating of your heart. Not every day can be an intense, wonder-filled visionary experience. I've tried living that way, believe me. The candle flame burns so quickly. But you can wake up, be glad you are alive, and face your day and the tasks before you with a desire to make the most out of what you're working on, doing, touching, saying.

You are here to live and to experience being human, so quit hiding. You may get hurt, yes. You may feel pain; we all do. It's part of this process, this journey we have embarked on. We cannot grow without stretching, and growth brings sorrow along with joy, the pain of loss and of saying good-bye, and, at the same time, transcendence over our fears and limitations. Growth offers us the chance to integrate the myriad facets of ourselves, to discover our inner passion and to push ourselves as far as we can.

What good are our talents, skills, and imagination if we do not use them? What good is the love in our hearts if we hide it in fear of rejection, in fear of pain? What good is having a body if we do not enjoy the feel of it? And in that enjoyment, yes, we will have days when we weep and wonder why we're going through the journey, why we're bothering. There is no escape from experiencing the downs of the cycle as well as the ups, but the adventure, the benefits, far outweigh the pain. Even when we are ridiculed and laughed at, we must have that steel core, that place of power within ourselves where we know our own direction and our own worth, where we can let the insults, slights, and taunts slide off like melted butter.

When we use our bodies, the pain will be there. Motion on muscles that have been atrophying for some time will hurt at first. Our bodies will resist. So we have to learn to transcend the pain, to revel in it, to immerse ourselves in it and come out the other side, and when we reach that place of transcendence, we soar. The endorphin rush alone is worth the effort, but once our bodies realize that we mean business, that we are going to make them move in whatever way we can, they fall into line and our energy level goes up, our eyes sparkle, we feel better, and we radiate with life.

When we are in our bodies, when we ground ourselves not only in our thoughts but our human-ness, we integrate the carnal and the cerebral, much like the god Pan, who represents the finer aspects of humanity—music and dance, and the carnal, lustful joy we are capable of experiencing. Only when we integrate these two sides of ourselves do we become whole.

When we feel good in our bodies, when we are secure in our accomplishments, when we embrace our existence with passion, then our beauty emerges from the inside and radiates through our exterior.

We shine, we soar…we live.

CHAPTER TWO

From the Inside Out: Nutrition to Clothing

What do you think would happen
if women stopped hating their bodies?

—Jane Hirschmann and Carol Munter,
When Women Stop Hating Their Bodies

WHY DISCUSS THIS AT ALL?

What do nutrition, weight, beauty, and grooming have to do with sex, the Divine, and loving your body? On the off chance that you don't see the connection, allow me to explain.

Our sexuality, on both physical and mystical levels, ties in with how healthy we feel, as well as how we view ourselves when we look in the mirror. If we keep ourselves well fed, if we exercise with a focus on health, if we adopt the attitude that we look great, our sexual energy will be much higher, and we will be more comfortable in our bodies when we interact with others. This allows us to stop worrying about things like "what do I look like, what are they thinking of me, how do I feel right now?" and keeps our focus on our energy. So these subjects, while seemingly peripheral, are vital considerations when we approach the connection of body and spirit.

A NOTE TO MY MALE READERS

I hope that you men who are reading this will bear with me through this chapter, much of which seems focused on women. Please remember how much emphasis is put on women's looks, how we are conditioned to pay attention to our shape, our size, our smell, our hair—everything you can imagine. Sometimes grooming is fun, and this is the way it should be. Other times, an intense scrutiny of the body can be terrifying to the point of causing despair.

So this chapter tends to focus a bit more on the female of the species, though I hope some of it will touch men's hearts. I enjoy the company of men but won't pretend to know what it's like to *be* male. However, since I *am* a woman, I hope to help my male readers better understand the female psyche so that we can deepen our levels of mutual understanding.

NUTRITION

While every body reacts differently to food, with specific nutritional requirements, depending on weight, health, allergies, etc., there are some basic building blocks that the majority of people need to some degree to maintain their health.

Perhaps this is elementary, but it is amazing how many people do not understand the revised concept of the food groups pyramid. Remember, your body may need different levels of each food group, but the USDA has revised the food guide pyramid as follows:

Daily Requirements for the Average Adult
- Vegetables: 3–5 servings
- Fruits: 2–4 servings
- Milk, cheese, yogurt: 2–3 servings
- Bread, cereal, rice, pasta: 6–11 servings

- Meat, poultry, fish, beans, eggs, nuts: 2–3 servings
- Fats, oils, sweets: eat sparingly
- Water: 8 glasses a day, at least

On a personal level, I adjust my eating habits according to how my body reacts. I don't handle complex carbohydrates very well, so with my doctor's approval, I eat very few of these. Conversely, my body needs more protein than carbohydrates and so I consume more meat, chicken, fish, and dairy. I also have a higher fruit intake. I have a diagnosed allergy to wheat, so I eliminate all wheat products (and believe me, that is no easy task).

You have to make allowances, depending on the needs of your family. My husband, a Type 1 diabetic, must follow a regimen of diet and exercise to stay healthy and safe. Use the food pyramid as a guideline and adjust it according to your specific needs and your doctor's orders. But remember: if you put low-octane fuel in your body, you won't perform in peak condition. You can't exist on a diet of pizza and cookies and expect to feel healthy.

Skipping breakfast leads to a heavier dinner, which you won't have time to digest properly if you eat it too late in the day. When you don't eat breakfast, your energy level will dip dramatically at mid-morning. If you eat a late dinner, your sleep won't be as restful. By spacing several smaller meals evenly throughout the day, your blood sugar will stay steady and so will your moods.

Even after years of practice in the Craft, after research and study and some common sense, even those who are advanced in their spiritual studies can end up doing something stupid. Last year, I deliberately got myself addicted to caffeine. I heard it speeded up metabolism and I thought, wow, it's also an appetite suppressant. Great! So I started drinking mochas. Now, I love mochas. I don't love coffee, don't even like the taste of it, but add chocolate and I'm a happy camper. Well, going on the theory that if a little buzz is fun, a lot more buzz would be better, I proceeded to increase my intake. I went from drinking one double espresso mocha per day to as many as eight shots of espresso with chocolate syrup and no milk. I cut down on my water intake. I couldn't figure out why I was so short-tempered, so lethargic when the caffeine buzz dropped, why I couldn't sleep most of the night, and why my skin was breaking out.

After a few months I mentioned this to my friend Patrick. He told me, "You twit, caffeine slows down the metabolism. It may stimulate the nerves, but it won't heighten your metabolic rate." He then proceeded calmly and snidely to tell me to cut down on my consumption of espresso, to start eating again (I was eating one meal a day), and eat more than I had before. I just had to make sure most of the food I was eating was healthy.

So I tried decaf, but couldn't take it without the buzz. However, I did manage to slow down to four shots of espresso a day. I increased my water intake and after a week, found myself hungry again. I was able to think clearly and was more focused. I also swallowed my pride when I had to tell Patrick he was right. Of course, he won't let me forget it. We have a love/hate relationship and admitting either one of us is right is never easy. But I had to face it: eating more food, healthier food, made me feel better once I was used to it again.

Check out the fads and do your research. Crash diets never helped anyone, and they do slow down your metabolism. If you have a food allergy, avoid that food entirely rather than playing chicken with it. Some food allergies can kill: others produce extreme discomfort. If your doctor tells you to reduce your cholesterol level, listen. Diet plays an integral part in how you feel and carry yourself, even how your hair and skin look. Eat healthy foods in moderation, enjoy what you eat, and don't let yourself become terrified of food. Drink at least eight glasses of water a day to flush out your system and to keep you from getting dehydrated. Take your vitamins and don't pop diet pills, which will only destroy the work you are trying to accomplish.

DIETING: THE MONSTER IN THE MIRROR

Look in the mirror. Sigh. Turn away in disgust. Cry. This routine is all too familiar for so many women I know. I've been there. But face it, people, diets don't work. Ninety-five percent of all those who attempt to diet don't succeed and most end up angry at themselves and at fate. Geneticists are now pinpointing genes that can account for body size. It seems that we have a predetermined setpoint that our bodies naturally gravitate to. Every person's body is different in this regard. You may be able to diet so that your setpoint is lowered, but chances are you'll have a hard time holding yourself there.

Another relatively new discovery is the important part exercise plays in the shape, size, and health of our bodies. The days are gone when people counted the calories in a doughnut and then walked X-amount of miles to work them off. Now we know that exercise and lean body muscle speed up metabolism, and metabolism can control weight. If you work out three times a week, twenty minutes per session, you will find your clothes fitting better, your health improving, and your attitude shifting. You won't have to worry then about your eating habits as long as you try to maintain a healthy and balanced diet.

Health, rather than the number on the scale or dress size, is becoming the focus for a number of women. For men, health, rather than appearance, has always been the focus, though that has shifted in recent years, too. We now know that *fat* and *fit* are not mutually exclusive. You can be larger than average and have blood pressure and cholesterol levels that are normal, and you most likely don't eat more than your thin counterparts. You can be fat and dance; you can be plump and swim; you can be buxom and incredibly sensuous. You can be large and be successful. Of course, now and then health risks will indicate that you need to lose weight. Always get a second opinion, and consider your options carefully.

If you still want or need to lose weight, your best course of action is to eat sensibly, attune your intake to your body's needs, and increase your exercise. Statistics show that those who have the most success in losing weight and keeping it off have developed their own system of doing so, tailored to their needs, tastes, and bodies. They have managed to come up with a plan they can live with, rather than focusing on short-term results. They've also lost weight slowly.

Even if you decide to lose weight, you must learn to love yourself and be happy with who you are. Don't support the diet industry by giving into the diet centers' ads. They thrive on repeat business; they live for your "failures."

Are you tempted to try those new drugs coming on the market? Remember Redux and Fen Phen? Do you really want to be a human guinea pig and end up potentially developing life-threatening conditions from side effects? Remember, if you put healthy food into your mouth, you'll be much better off than if you deplete yourself of the building blocks that support your life.

You also run the risk, if you allow yourself to be sucked in by the diet mentality, of developing an eating disorder. Anorexia, bulimia, binge eating: all of these are dangerous to your system and devastating to your psyche. If you think you already have an eating disorder, I beg you, get help. These conditions are life-threatening and almost impossible to get rid of without counseling. There are people out there to help you. Any crisis clinic can help direct you to resources within your community. Unfortunately, many people, most of them women, who develop eating disorders don't see what's happening to them. They have a distorted sense of body image and cannot see how they are destroying themselves. If you know someone with an eating disorder, talk to them and offer to help them find help.

MY BATTLE WITH DIETING AND SELF-ESTEEM

I remember looking at myself in the mirror, loathing my image. I couldn't imagine what I might possess that would save me. All my talent and skills seemed pitiful compared to one thing: I was fat. Not ugly, but fat. And this, as we all know, is a supreme sin in our society. I had great hair, good features, I loved my dark eyes and hair and pale skin, but I wasn't thin.

As a child, I was on a constant diet. The only thing beyond my writing, the only other thing that mattered in my world, was that I was fat. Now, when I look at pictures of myself from that period, I see that I was chubby, not huge. I grew up in a house where weight was a pre-occupation. My bloodline runs to heavy women, sturdy mountain women. Cherokee and Irish, built for stamina and endurance rather than speed.

As I grew up, genetics weren't considered a factor in size, except in old wives' tales. Only will power mattered. If you were weak, you gained weight. If you were strong, you lost it. And beauty was reserved for the thin. Twiggy was in vogue; Mama Cass was out of favor.

My struggle began when I was eleven years old and didn't stop until I reached my thirties. I tried all the diets: eight hundred calories a day; Dr. Stillman's all-meat diet; five hundred calories a day; the lettuce and tomato diet; TOPS weight loss program; fasts for a week at a time; give up this food; give up that food; eat only three meals a day; eat what you want as long as it's only one bowl of combined foods; starve yourself; vegetarianism; Susan Powter's non-diet fat-free diet. I tried everything except bulimia and no doubt that's because I hadn't heard of it. I saved that one for later on in my late twenties.

I lost weight—twenty-five pounds on the protein diet—until I got sick. On the low-calorie and the low/no-protein diets, low blood sugar gave me massive headaches. My metabolism slowed down due to too little food and I gained weight. I didn't understand—no one seemed to—that if you go below a certain number of calories, your body shuts down and you begin to utilize food in a more efficient way. I hated exercise because I was forced to do it, almost as a punishment for my size.

When I look back at my photos I think, if I'd been left alone and hadn't gone on those diets, I would have evened out. I'd be larger than the average person, but not the way I eventually became. And if some of the current medical findings had been known then, it would have helped too.

For one thing, I'm allergic to wheat. A number of people are finding that allergies to food affect their bodies in odd ways. There is now evidence that some people are insulin-sensitive; because carbohydrates produce insulin in some people and insulin acts as an anabolic agent, carbohydrate intake can prevent people from losing weight. For example, on the low/no-fat diet, when I was eating less than 15 grams of fat a day and massive quantities of carbohydrates, I lost weight for a week or two and then began to pile it back on. This can lead to insulin resistance, which can supposedly bring on adult-onset diabetes. Therefore, low blood sugar can turn into its opposite.

After I discovered that my wheat allergy had grown worse, I accepted the inevitable and gave up eating wheat. I also took in fewer complex carbohydrates and my weight stopped creeping up. I've actually lost some weight, even though I presently eat more fat and my calorie count has not decreased. You see, each body is unique, and responds to food, as to all substances, uniquely.

When I was with my ex, while he did not belittle my looks or my weight, neither did he support my struggle for self-acceptance emotionally. And he actively sought to interfere with my creativity by telling me, "If you are successful as an author, I will have to leave you." When we parted ways, I developed a short-term bout with bulimia. It was easy to do: all I had to do was visualize losing my dinner, and I did. Then I thought, why eat dinner if I'm just going to lose it? So I stopped eating dinner, ate only a small lunch, and no breakfast. And why not? I had heard all my life that men wouldn't want me because I was fat.

About that time, my therapist prescribed antidepressants. I reluctantly began taking them and within a few weeks was eating and sleeping again. My bout with eating disorders ended. However, I realize I will always have the potential to fall back into bulimia, so I watch myself. After the antidepressants took hold, I began to even out, to view the world through less agonized eyes. I realized I was tired of feeling like an outcast. I was tired of apologizing for who I was, for my looks or my brains. I was tired of dieting and becoming even larger, and I was fed up with feeling embarrassed. I realized that I was through tearing myself down just to boost someone else's ego. I decided then and there that I would no longer make any unnecessary compromises. I must admit I had help along the way, and I don't think I could have reached this point without a few wonderful milestones.

A few months later, I met a young man. He was twenty-one years old, eight years younger than me. I thought he just wanted to be friends until he came over to visit, grabbed a brush to brush my hair, and then leaned me back in his arms and kissed me. We spent a few wonderful, sexy, and passionate months together before I decided that we had nothing in common except the bedroom and, as nice as he was, the relationship wouldn't work. I gently let him go, much happier and forever grateful to this young Georgia boy who helped me feel like a desirable woman again.

After that I found my way into the local Pagan community and for the first time in years began making friends. Suddenly I found myself the recipient of quite a lot of male attention. My self-esteem rose even further, and I began to see that the lies I'd been fed about fat women being unattractive were just that: lies. Then, when I met Samwise, I was amazed when he fell head over heels in love with me in less than a week. At one point, he took my hand and said, "I can't understand why you aren't with anyone. You could have any man you want."

REKINDLING YOUR CONNECTION WITH FOOD

If you are used to denying yourself permission to eat what you want, this may prove to be a difficult exercise. It was for me at first. I cannot eat everything I want because of my wheat allergy. But once I refused to eat the things that hurt my body, I can and do eat anything and everything else that I desire without guilt. By allowing myself this freedom, I keep my cravings to a minimum and no longer find myself bingeing on any food.

Go to your cupboards. Taking other family members' likes and dislikes into account, remove anything you purchased because it was supposed to be good for you. If you like it, that's fine, keep it. If you don't, get rid of it. For years, I bought rice cakes, but when I finally admitted that I don't like them, I quit buying them.

Next, examine the food you are keeping. Is there a preponderance of junk food in your cupboards? It's fine to eat Twinkies twice a week, or even once a day, but you need to make sure you are fueling your body with good, healthy food, too. Instead of skipping meals and then snacking your way through the junk food aisles later, buy the best-quality food you can afford and make nice dinners for yourself and your family.

If you don't have time to cook every day, buy the ingredients and once every two weeks, cut, chop, cook, and freeze. Stir-fries take only a few minutes to prepare if you have everything cut up in advance. A beef stew can be made in quantity and frozen in individual servings and microwaved before dinnertime. Make a list of foods you like that are healthy and taste good, and then go shopping. Fill your cupboards. Chances are you'll eat better if you have the food available.

Take the time to set a nice table at least twice a week. If you are living with someone, it can be a romantic and relaxing way to connect with that person. If you on your own, treat yourself like an honored guest in your home. Buy flowers, candles, a pretty vase, placemats. Don't have much money? Your local thrift shop will usually have some lovely dishes, some of them antiques, for pennies.

Make your meals a time to converse, or think about the day. Turn off the television, turn on the music or turn it off for blessed silence, and take a few minutes out from your hectic schedule. You will find yourself appreciating the fuel that goes into your bodies more and digesting your food better because you have eaten it in peace without rushing.

Do you have problems giving yourself permission to eat certain foods you've outlawed? Many diet centers use that term to refer to foods not on their eating plans, creating the impression that some foods are inherently bad. No food, in and of itself, is evil. Your body may react to it in a way that makes it unsuitable for you, but the food itself should not be considered bad.

To counter these feelings of guilt, try one of the following methods.

Freedom to Eat Visualization
Sit in a quiet place and relax. Focus inward and see yourself sitting at a table with a clean place setting in front of you. Imagine that your

favorite foods are on the table and that you can have anything you want. Are there any foods that you tell yourself not to touch, though there is no medical reason for doing so? If so, put a small portion of one of these foods on your plate. Now look at it, see it for what it is—simply food, with no good or bad connotations. If you eat it, know that you will not be a bad person; you will simply be eating one of a number of foods available to us. Now see yourself picking up your fork or spoon and taking a bite. Imagine how it tastes. If you feel guilty, say to yourself, "Food carries no moral judgment." When you feel okay about eating this food, try another that you've banned from your diet. Repeat this exercise daily, until you are comfortable with the idea of eating these foods in moderation to satisfy your hunger.

Fire Spell for Freedom from Guilt

For this spell, you will need a piece of blank paper, a pen, a bowl with a thin layer of salt in it, and a red candle.

Cut the piece of paper into strips. On each strip, write down an attitude that you carry toward diet and food, one you'd like to get rid of. For example, "I release myself from feeling guilty when I eat chocolate," or "I release the need to count every calorie that goes in my mouth." When you have assembled your pile of paper strips, cast a Circle, call the Elements,[1] and light the candle.

Invoke Kwan Yin, the goddess of mercy, blessings, and grace. Say:

Kwan Yin, Gracious Jade Goddess, please hear my call and answer. Look to my rites, help me heal my vision of myself and release those attitudes that hamper my evolution. You are a goddess of mercy and healing, and I ask for your blessing. So mote it be.

Now take up each strip of paper, read aloud what you've written on it, and light it with the candle. Drop the burning strip into the bowl and go onto the next one. When you are done, cool the ashes and wash them away down the sink into the sewer system. If you have a septic tank, put the ashes on the ground. Then smudge[2] yourself with either sage or frankincense and let the candle burn out. Always keep water near you in case of an accident when you are working with fire magick.

BASIC SKIN CARE

Your skin is the largest organ on your body and is composed of two layers: the epidermis and the dermis. The epidermis is the upper layer and includes the surface. The dermis lies below, and contains the blood vessels, oil, sweat glands, nerves, etc. What you eat affects your skin and any approach to skin care has to take into account dietary factors.

Basic Skin Care Hints

- If you are vitamin-deficient, if your diet mainly consists of junk, or if you don't get enough sleep, your skin will tell.
- If you have serious acne, consult a physician. They are discovering that it's caused by factors other than diet, and there are a number of medications out there to treat it now.
- Keep your skin protected from the sun with at least a 30 SPF sunscreen.
- Gently cleanse your skin twice a day, and then apply a good moisturizer.
- When you use cosmetics, thoroughly remove them before you go to bed.
- When you choose a moisturizer, remember that, unlike perfume, an inexpensive one may work just as well as one of the high-priced brands.

- Do not pick or prod at blackheads and pimples. Yes, yes, I know how hard this is and all I can say is try not to do it—you could push the infection deeper and leave a scar.
- I shave my arms as well as my legs, to let my tattoos show up better. Shaved skin needs a good cream to keep it supple and protected. Don't forget this step after you shave.
- When shaving your legs or any other part of your body, stick to a razor and gel rather than chemicals that can burn you. Change the blade often and don't leave it in a moist place where bacteria can grow. If you nick yourself, a stipple stick will take care of the cut quickly with a minimum of fuss.
- Try not to rest your chin on your hand all the time. The pressure can produce boils, pimples, and discoloration.
- Wrinkles are more likely to happen if you smoke, when you frown, when you don't release the stress you accumulate in your body. Take an afternoon to assess your stress levels and determine what you can do to reduce tension in your life.
- One of the best ways to make your skin beautiful is to drink plenty of water. Drink at least eight glasses a day.

BASIC HAIR CARE

Oh, no, another Bad Hair Day! The phrase is part and parcel of our language now. We identify with our hair, we agonize over bad cuts and styles. Hair is viewed as sexy, as embodying power. Even the lack of hair speaks loud and clear: with men, it often signifies strength (e.g., Yul Brynner), sometimes growing old; with women, the loss of hair is usually embarrassing. You want to find a cut that works for you, that you are comfortable with, and that you can maintain. I have been with my stylist for five years and trust him more than I trust anyone except my tattooist (that is, when I am looking at people who provide me with professional services).

Hair is composed of keratin, the same substance in our nails. The hair we see on our body is dead, but the hair follicle is alive. When the follicles die, we see hair loss.

We tease it, we dye it, we perm it, we straighten it, we rat it, and we coat it with layers of hair spray and chemicals. Is it any wonder our poor hair breaks and splits at the ends? Dyes, excessive heat, excessive or rough brushing, and harsh detergents can all damage the cuticle of our hair, which surrounds the cortex and hair shaft. Then we attempt to rectify this damage with products that nourish and moisturize our scalp and locks.

As with our skin and our bodies, if we do not nourish the inside, we will not see results on the outside. Inadequate protein and caloric intake account for thinning or loss of hair. Extreme stress can affect it, as can hormonal imbalances (such as found during pregnancy or with PMS). Not eating enough fat? Expect your hair to dry out. You have dandruff (seborrhea)? Have you tried monitoring your level of stress? Have you been sick, or have you neglected to wash the shampoo and conditioner completely out of your hair? For mild cases of dandruff, a specially formulated shampoo can help. For more extreme conditions, consult a physician.

Shampoos, Conditioners, and Brushing

When you buy shampoo and conditioner, check to see how your scalp reacts to different brands. For example, one brand makes my skin break out and then scab. Shampoos consist primarily of two ingredients: detergent and water. The detergent cleans your hair, removing oil and dirt and pollutants from both scalp and hair shafts. The water dilutes the detergent.

Some shampoos include other ingredients:

- Agents to thicken the shampoo and reduce wateriness and to help the detergent lather up.
- Preservatives to prevent bacteria from building up.
- Vitamins, which are for the most part useless. They just add to the price of the shampoo. Most vitamins are too large to enter the hair shaft, and since the hair is essentially dead, it cannot be "nourished." However, there is some evidence that vitamin E may provide an antioxidizing effect, and Panthenol may be able to penetrate the hair shaft and strengthen the hair.
- Herbs for fragrance. They can have positive effects on the scalp and some effect on hair coloration.
- Non-herbal fragrances to make the shampoo smell good.
- Balsam, a resin that adds volume by coating the hair shaft.
- Dyes to make the shampoo look good.

There are shampoos for different hair types. I use the ones for color-treated hair since I dye my hair regularly. I find that this is a guess-and-go game. Opt for sample sizes until you find something you like; change your brand every few months to avoid buildup; and make sure to wash all the shampoo out of your hair.

Conditioners are formulated to leave a residue on your hair through the positive/negative charge/polarity of your hair which coats and protects your hair shaft. A good conditioner will also act as a detangler. Conditioners can be either oil-based or oil-free. You should make your decision based on what shape your hair is in. A deep conditioner, used weekly or monthly, tends to have a smaller molecular structure and will penetrate the hair more easily than daily-use conditioners.

Once again, try various brands until you discover what works for your hair type. Conditioner is especially important if you use a blow dryer, dye or perm your hair, or live in an area full of air pollutants.

When you brush your hair, following these hints can make a world of difference in how your hair looks and reacts:

- Don't brush one hundred strokes a day; this will break your hair. Brush until it's untangled and styled.
- Don't brush your hair while it's wet. You will run the risk of stretching the hair shaft and damaging it.
- Look for rounded-tipped bristles when you choose a brush.
- Use combs with wide teeth rather than narrow teeth.
- Do brush your hair once or twice a day.
- Give yourself regular scalp massages. This stimulates the blood flow, helps prevent dandruff, and reduces tension.

Hair Dyes

There are four primary types of hair color.

Level 1 hair color, or *temporary hair color,* lasts from one to six shampoos and primarily coats the hair shaft. The majority of level 1 colors contain no peroxides and are often used for special occasions or to experiment with a specific color.

Level 2 hair color, or *semi-permanent hair color,* lasts from six to twenty-four shampoos. Darker shades of dyes may stain lighter colored hair for a long period of time. This is a very common type of hair dye, used by those who wish to cover small patches of gray, to enhance their own hair color, or to give a slight tint to their hair. Some people may have an allergic reaction to this dye, so do a patch test according to the directions.

Level 3 hair color, or *permanent hair color,* lasts a long time. It may fade a bit but generally the only way to change it is with another permanent color. Remember, if you go darker than your natural shade, you may have to bleach it to get back to the lighter shades. This hair color contains strong chemicals, bleaches, peroxides, and dyes and can cause allergic reactions, so make sure to do a patch test, following the directions included with the dye.

Henna and other *vegetable dyes* make up the fourth type of hair color. I've heard varying reports on whether henna can hurt hair; the consensus seems to be that if metallic oxides are added (and they often are) to alter the color of the vegetable powder, the powder may rough up your hair. I used henna for years and though I did love some of the effects, I finally switched over to commercial dyes. The results are much more predictable, they cover gray better, and the dyes are much less messy than working with henna powder.

Coloring your hair can change not only how *you* feel about yourself, but how others feel about you. Studies have been done on how people react to the same person as a brunette, blonde, and redhead. It is interesting to note the qualities our culture connects with hair color. I have been every shade of red, blue-black, and just about every shade of brown. The only color I haven't wanted to play with (indeed, have had nightmares of being) is blonde, because it would clash with my coloring. My favorite hair color is burgundy-plum, though I have to admit, I look better with dark chocolate brown hair, which accentuates my pale skin and dark eyes.

People, even my husband, have asked me why I don't let my hair grow out to its natural color. Well, I came to silver early and have quite a bit of it sprinkled through my hair. I tell these people I'm just not ready—I'm not in the Crone stage in my life; and I feel much more comfortable with dark, dark hair. Silver will be beautiful when I'm ready, but not now.

Tips on coloring your hair:

- Use quality products and follow directions. You want to keep your hair, not lose it. Always do a patch test and a strand test.
- Use a conditioner every time you shampoo.
- Before doing "extreme coloring," make sure you're ready to handle the emotional changes that come with changing your looks in such a drastic manner. You may find yourself freaking out, or you may suddenly find yourself acting like a different person. Are you ready for that?

Moon-Mother Hair Spell for Women

You can call in the power of the moon and her femininity as part of your beauty ritual. During the time from the New Moon to the Full Moon, sit near a window each night while wearing a moonstone necklace. Brush your hair gently while repeating:

Moon Mother, Moon Mother, glowing down on me,
Let my beauty radiate, shine for all to see.

During the phases from Full to New, wear a black onyx or obsidian necklace each night and brush your hair while chanting:

Moon Mother, Moon Mother, Dark Lady, look to me,
Bathe me in your secret light, cloaked in mystery.

COSMETICS

Lipstick, rouge, perfume, eye shadow, mascara, foundation, nail polish, eyeliner...the list goes on and I love them all! I find playing with cosmetics a meditation, and as long as I don't reach the point where I feel as if I have to wear them to be beautiful, or I can't go out of the house without them, I think I'm doing fine.

Cosmetics were and are used in religious ceremonies and ritual to alter the body and to symbolize the body's connection with spirit. It is also thought by some anthropologists that when applying lipstick, women have a subconscious recollection of our more primitive roots. The genitals on our primate relatives often turn bright red when the female is ready for mating, and the application of red lipstick is thought to have a connection with this. Artificial beauty marks were used centuries ago to cover up scars left from the bubonic plague and smallpox.

Today, especially within the American modern-primitives subculture, it is acceptable for men to use cosmetics, whether or not they are gender-benders. With the advent of warehouse-style pharmacies and drug stores and with the massive corporations appealing to vanity, the choices are almost unlimited.

My only complaints with people's focus on beauty products are these:

- The media uses a woman's fear of growing older as an incentive to buy the newest products from Company X or Corporation Z. Cosmetics become a weapon against age, thus promoting ageism.
- Women (and I say women here, because my primary concerns are about women's issues) are being brainwashed into believing they can't be beautiful without these products.
- Exorbitant prices are attached to a lot of these products because of the designer name or the packaging. With perfume, you do get what you pay for. I am willing to pay a high price for perfume because I know how expensive some of the ingredients can be and nothing smells worse than cheap perfume. But with most makeup, there isn't that much difference between the expensive and cheaper brands.

The point I am trying to make is that you should have fun with cosmetics, play with them, revel in them, use them for ritual, experiment with them, but don't rely on them to create the inner you. All the outer beauty in the world isn't going to build the person within. However, if you are lovely on the inside, but you feel plain on the outside, a good makeover can make a world of difference in your perspective, and when you see yourself differently, others will notice and they too will alter their behavior.

Some Tips on Purchasing and Using Cosmetics

- Every six months clean your makeup case and get rid of any cosmetics which seem old. Look for signs of mold or bacteria growth. If you haven't replaced your mascara or eyeliner in the past six months, do so.
- Keep tubes of lipstick in the refrigerator and then remove an hour before use.
- With perfume, you get what you pay for. Imitations of designer perfumes are easy to spot by their pungent and sometimes harsh scents. Buy the best perfume you can afford. You can buy good six to seven dollar tubes of lipstick, but don't waste your money on poor-quality fragrance. Buy the real thing, or buy essential oils.
- Get your color chart done at a free makeover. Every mall with a Bon Marché or a Nordstrom's will offer free makeovers. Take advantage of the favor. You may not like what they do, but you can get valuable advice on what colors go best with your skin. For example, I look very good with the dark burgundy tones and the purplish dark reds, but get me near true red or orange red and I look awful. I look great in emerald greens and bronze, but coffee colors and taupe? Nope. Experiment and see what

you like and what looks good on you. If necessary, find a compromise between the two.

• Don't buy products that are tested on animals.

The Hathor Beauty Spell

Hathor was the Egyptian goddess of women, strength, and beauty. I often invoked her when I applied my makeup every day. Buy a candle, burgundy or beeswax, and into it carve this rune, which is a symbol for Hathor.

On the other side, carve your name and the words: "beauty," "strength," and "passion." Anoint the candle with olive oil and put it in a beautiful candleholder. Each day that you decide to wear cosmetics, light the candle before putting on your makeup. Put on music that strikes a sensual chord, and before you begin your routine, say:

Hathor, Lady of the Desert, Goddess of Women, I call to thee.
From your deserts of Egypt, look down to me.
Hear me, Hathor, and attend my rite.
Let my inner beauty shine with radiant light.
Let me be strong and capable, gentle and loving, brilliant and wise.
Let all these qualities shine forth from my body, from my eyes.

When you are finished, snuff the candle and save it until the next day.

In conclusion, to enhance your body, treat it with reverence. Decorating the skin is the same as decorating your temple within. There's nothing wrong with this as long as we remember that our spirit flows from our hearts, our souls, and our minds, not from our faces.

---

1. See appendix 1: Magickal Rites and Elemental Charts.
2. Ibid.

CHAPTER THREE

Impressions and Attitudes

A lovely lady, garmented in light
From her own beauty.

—Percy Bysshe Shelley, "The Witch of Atlas"

Want to make a dynamite impression? Want to shine, glow, and radiate? How you walk, how you hold yourself, how you move—these affect how people look at you, and how you feel about yourself. If you want to enter a room and make heads turn, not just because of your looks, but because of your energy, pay attention to the following:

- Stride as if you own the world, but not as if the world owes you a living.
- Move as if you know every secret action your body can make, but don't make this so obvious that everyone can see you without first delving into your mysteries.
- When you shake someone's hand, grip it firmly and meet that person's gaze.
- Know that you are worth every drop of attention you get, but also know when to step back from the spotlight.

Poise can make the difference between getting a job and not getting it, between attracting a lover and being alone, between wincing as you pass a mirror or smiling because you know you are strong in your own sense of self. Samwise told me the very first thing that attracted him to me was the way I held myself—he says I have a regal posture, which told him I value myself.

Hand in hand with self-confidence, *poise* is part of the way we express our self-esteem through our bodies. It's not simply a matter of elegance, correcting your posture, or learning how to shake hands— poise truly comes down to being comfortable in your body and being comfortable with yourself. If you appreciate and value yourself, if you know that you matter, it shows in your actions, in your words, and in your eyes.

People respond to body language. If you always walk hunched over and refuse to meet people's eyes, if you act as if you are ashamed of yourself, people will mirror this. Self-loathing leads to being dismissed or loathed by others.

Think about it. You walk into a store and ask about a product and the clerk tells you, "Oh, it's not really that good. You think it's pretty, but look closer. See? There's a scratch there, and a blemish there. There are other models that can do more for you than this one." Would you buy the object in question? Probably not. Now transfer that scenario to your own life. When you act as if you have nothing to offer and as if you do not value yourself, how can you expect anyone to treat you with respect and admiration? If they do, chances are you'll brush off their compliments. Self-degradation can become a habit and can make you sound like you're wallowing in self-pity. People who whimper about their faults and seem to crave constant shoring up are not people you want to know—they aren't attractive.

What most people fail to realize is that while appreciative gazes, comments, and reactions can all help heighten our self-confidence, we must have that confidence established in the first place in order for this added attention to ring true in our hearts. Otherwise we soak up the energy, the compliments, feed on them for a time, and then once again find ourselves bereft and needing more. We become emotional and psychic vampires, gaining all our self-confidence from others instead of cultivating it from within.

Most of us have met people who brush off our compliments, who are self-deprecating at every chance. Tell them they look nice and they'll say, "No, no…." Tell them they've got a lovely voice and they'll say, "It's the song that sounded good." Tell them they are smart and they'll say, "I made a lucky guess."

After a time, this behavior starts to grate on our nerves and wears us down. Soon we begin to avoid people who constantly drag us down with their tortured self-doubts and inner demons. We cringe when we hear them on the phone, we go out of our way to find a reason not to drop by. They need us too much and they don't ever have time to discuss our problems or needs because they are always focused on their own insecurities.

Some people seem to relish their angst, perhaps because for a time they get attention that way. But in the long run, touting their list of faults, problems, and reasons why they can't accept a compliment leads to losing friends. This type of person is labor-intensive because they require high maintenance emotionally.

It is true that at times we all have periods of doubting certain aspects of ourselves. There's no avoiding this. However, if we can keep these aspects in proportion to everything else, if we can find a balance and see both what is exquisite about us as well as what needs work, then we are going to find a way to radiate our beauty.

Now, no one wants to be around a perfect person, but it's always nice to be with someone who sparkles with the knowledge that she or he is special. When you recognize your positive qualities and enhance them, it allows you to see and point out the good in others, because you aren't threatened by the successes another might have. Our insecurity about ourselves leads to our deprecation of others.

CARRIAGE

Carriage is an old-fashioned, though not yet archaic, term for how we carry our bodies. While all grace springs from the inside, we can enhance how we express this inner beauty with how we comport ourselves. Not only does your posture show how you feel about yourself, it also affects your health. Poor posture contributes to the incorrect alignment of your spine, to headaches, stomachaches, and to inadequate or uncomfortable sleep.

First, you must try to feel out your body and examine why you aren't standing in a straight but comfortable position.

- Your spine must be in alignment. A good chiropractor makes all the difference.
- Exercise will change the way you move and stand. I'm not talking about jogging or hardcore bodybuilding, but flowing movements such as dancing, yoga, and walking.[1]
- Proper-fitting shoes can make a big difference. If you teeter in heels but persist in wearing them, you will not be graceful, just awkward. Similarly, if your shoes are too tight or too loose, you won't be able to move with poise and confidence.
- If you lead a sedentary life, proper chairs and footrests are necessary. I write a good portion of the day and my back would be in agony if I hadn't bought a comfortable desk chair. I'm so short that most chairs leave my feet unable to touch the floor, so I either wear heels while working or use a footrest.

- Stress plays a big part in how we stand and move. Even just mild, day-to-day tension can eat away at our bodies and erode our confidence. Take a few minutes several times a day to perform shoulder rolls, neck rolls, and mild stretching in order to release that built-up tension. Yawning helps too.
- Pent-up sexual frustration and/or tension can cause our posture to tighten. We often pull back into ourselves and become more on edge if this continues for any length of time. If you have no sexual partner, learn to masturbate.[2] There is nothing wrong with masturbation, and most of the guilt we feel is derived from childhood, from our shame-based puritanical culture. There is a long history of autoerotism in sex magick, and unless your self-pleasuring interferes with your day-to-day life, don't worry about how often you masturbate.
- A good massage on a regular basis can make quite a difference in how your body feels and looks. Massage in and of itself can be a spiritual practice.
- We are often not taught how to walk or to sit so that we can present ourselves effectively and learn how to be graceful and forceful at the same time. You do not have to tiptoe around in a mincing way to be graceful. You can stride into a room and still be the most feminine woman there, or you can walk in with poise and serenity and exude masculinity. I learned how to walk, sit, and stand through being in theater. Acting classes and learning to direct taught me how to present myself and my actors on stage in their best possible light. Can't afford to take a class? Don't have access to one? Watch movies with sensual, attractive, magnetic characters. How do they move? Watch their body language. You can learn by imitation, though I suggest you find your own style. I do not walk with feminine, little steps; I

stride, I am firm of foot, and yet I do so in a way which totally fits my skirts and lingerie and high-heeled boots (when I'm not barefoot).

- Remember, good posture doesn't mean you are stiff as a board. Indicators of a good stance are shoulders that are back but not rigid, an upright head and eyes facing forward, stomach comfortably tucked back a bit, and knees ever-so-slightly bent to avoid strain. I used to find that wearing a backpack, evenly filled but not too heavy, did wonders for my posture. There are some very good yoga postures which help, too.

VOICE AND GREETINGS

I still don't care for my voice, but everyone always says they like it. I put it down to not being able to hear myself correctly and now I don't worry about it.

However, in the past, I found myself occasionally getting breathless in a way that made me choke off some of my words or stumble over the ends of sentences. I know that others have problems with speaking aloud, especially in public. Again, my theatrical background helped me, but there are also some effective simple exercises in diction and elocution. Proper breathing will help. If you breathe in a rhythmic and steady fashion, your expression will be smooth and your presentation will be natural and not forced.

Breathing in Rhythm

Loosen any tight clothing you are wearing. Stand in a relaxed, comfortable position. Take a slow, deep breath and slowly exhale. Roll your shoulders to the front, slowly and smoothly. Around and down, back and up. And again. Now roll your shoulders to the back, slowly and in a smooth motion. Around and down, forward and up. And again.

Roll your neck slowly and gently from left to right, touching chin to chest as you do so. Very gently stretch, but do not roll your head so that it hangs over your back. Now slowly and gently roll your head the other way, from right to left, touching your chin to your chest as you do so. Continue for a few moments until you've worked the kinks out of your neck and shoulders.

Now, take a slow (but not too deep) breath from your diaphragm.[3] As your lower abdomen expands, the incoming air should force your chest to rise. Hold for a count of four, then slowly exhale. Your diaphragm should contract as you breathe out. Hold for a count of four and then repeat. Practice this breath over a period of several weeks until you can rhythmically and slowly breathe this way for five minutes. Do *not* hyperventilate or you will run the risk of fainting.

When you are comfortable, try walking while breathing this way. See if you can keep your breath even and relaxed. Don't walk fast enough to speed up your respiration, just feel the breath synchronized with your movements.

Next, practice reading a passage aloud, pacing your words so they fall naturally with your breathing. If you notice yourself running out of air in the middle of a sentence, know you have to break it in a logical place.

If you work with this exercise enough, you'll find that you will become calmer and more comfortable in your daily life. The breath is everything, supercharged with *prana, chi,* life force, and all the other names it's known by. We do not breathe correctly in this country—we rush around, panicking, forgetting to take the breath into our lungs rather than just into our throats. Breath is life.

TONGUE TWISTER TIME

Find yourself getting tongue-tied and tripping over words? Remember as a child when you played tongue twister games? These are no mere children's games, they are valuable exercises and tools. We used them a lot during my acting classes. They are fun and really do help. The point behind these exercises is not to repeat the tongue twisters fast, the way we did when we were kids, but to say them evenly, navigating the sounds, and enunciating them clearly and rhythmically.

These chants are designed to build a person's confidence and ability in the spoken word. Begin slowly and focus on what you are doing. Feel how your tongue glides over the sounds. Some people have more difficulty making certain sounds than others; I myself pronounce certain words in the British fashion because it's easier on my lips and mouth. I pronounce laboratory *la-bor'-a-tory* rather than the American *lab'-ra-tory*. It is simply easier for my tongue to navigate the sounds.

After you have gotten comfortable practicing the tongue twisters, put them into motion—after all, we do talk when we walk. Walk in a circle, slow and evenly, while repeating the phrases. Gradually speed up your movements until you are walking at a good, but not hectic, pace. See if you can match the cadence of your words to the pace of your steps.

Here are some of the common tongue twisters we all grew up with and love—they are still wonderful practice pieces. I've thrown in a few new ones and some I learned in acting class. Repeat each phrase at least ten times.

Red leather, yellow leather.
You know you need unique New York.
Five corpulent porpoises.
Pick cherries at their peak or Pete will see the pips.

Beach bins are filled with field filler.
Alice asks for axes.
Two Witches watched two watches. Which Witch watched which watch?
Three fluffy feathers fell from Phoebe's flimsy fan.

READING ALOUD

Another wonderful way to get used to speaking is to read aloud. Read to your children, read to your significant other, read to your cat. Read everything—especially poetry. Drift into the characters, become them, take on their attributes, snarl when they do, shout when they do, laugh when they do, weep when they do. Let your voice mirror the voice of the words. If you read aloud for ten minutes a day, you will find yourself more comfortable speaking in public because your voice will become accustomed to prolonged use.

CHANTING

Now, I'm not going to say that everyone can become a good singer by practicing chanting. I am good with chants, but I will admit it—singing isn't one of my natural-born talents. Chanting has a long and established history for raising energy, focusing the will, and as in our case here, working the voice.

There's no reason why you can't practice chanting for poise and confidence while you are also expanding the range of your vocal cords. Unfortunately, I can't give you the music here. But you can create your own music for the chants. By singing them either in a Circle or by yourself, you will invite the energies embodied in their words into your life to work for you. Some of these chants can be used as affirmations as well.

When you are chanting, remember not to end the chant too soon. When you keep it going for more than five or six rounds, you will find yourself slipping into trance and your voice will grow stronger and your energy will rise.

Surf the wave, ride the crest
Life always works out for the best.

Let strength and beauty fill my life
Let sight be keen, wit be bright
Let fire burn within my heart
I balance the dance of light and dark.

Everything in my life works out more exquisitely than I plan it.

Fire burn, fire burn, fire burn bright
In the depths of the darkness, the dark of the night.
Fire burn, fire burn, fire burn bright
Set my heart ablaze, bathe me in your light.
Fire burn, fire burn, fire burn bright
Shake the shadows of the past, soar me to new heights.

You can create your own chants about any aspect of yourself you would like to see changed or strengthened, or use the above for general purposes. Remember when chanting to keep your voice at a resonant pitch; vocalize with strength and clarity, and remain sure of yourself.

GREETING PEOPLE

When we first meet people who shift their gaze away from ours or who shake our hand with a languid grip and mutter a hello, we tend either to view them with suspicion or wonder if they truly want to meet us.

Greetings vary from culture to culture. In some cultures, it is considered the height of bad manners to look someone in the eye; in others, like ours, refusing to make eye contact is regarded with suspicion. If you travel out of the country, be sure to study the people you are likely to meet. You do not want to make an error based on ignorance.

When you encounter someone new, you will generally want to project self-confidence and a "glad to meet you" face and manner. Some of those old courses in etiquette could stand people in good stead today. When you shake someone's hand, grip it firmly but not tightly. Men, allow a woman to offer to shake your hand first. If she chooses to forego the ritual, simply nod and smile as you greet her.

Keep your voice level and your eyes focused on the other person. Repeat his or her name as you shake hands—a good method for remembering it. The energy you project is the energy that people will read. If you come across as mousy and insecure, the other person will pick up on it and view you as such. This is especially important during job interviews. Statistics show that within thirty seconds, employers make up their minds about whether or not you have a chance for the job. Those thirty seconds are not spent focused on how nice you are or your skills, but on how you look, and more importantly, on how you present yourself.

CLOTHING

What you choose to wear tells a great deal about you. If you are comfortable in your clothes, you will act more comfortable. Find the style that works for you and keep your clothes neat and clean. Do not wear clothes that are too tight or clothes you won't be able to move in comfortably. It will look as if you are disguising the size you are.

I am most at home in long gauzy skirts and lingerie tops. I never wear trousers; I haven't in over twenty years. They just aren't me. If I felt more comfortable (bodywise) in leather miniskirts, I'd wear them, but they don't fit my current shape or my personal comfort. I wear more cosmetics and perfume than most of my friends do, but I don't layer it on, and there are many days I go completely without makeup. I almost always wear perfume. My husband, Samwise, wears jeans or pants, T-shirts, an occasional dress shirt, a leather jacket, but never ties or suits. They just don't fit his style. I have other friends who never climb out of jeans and still others who wear Versace all of the time.

If your style is true to you, if you don't try to force yourself into a style that doesn't work for you, if you don't let stereotypes determine what you wear, life should be easier for you.

Fat? You don't have to wear polyester or tents; you *can* look as sexy as you want. Rail thin? Really want to wear vertical stripes? Go ahead, it's your body and if you feel comfortable in your clothes, the energy will show through. Have you been told you look best in green but you are dying to wear red? Give it a try, see how you like it. Don't let the fashion magazines tell you what to do.

Generally, if you dress appropriately for the situation, keep your clothes clean and in good repair, and replace them when they're old, faded, or stained, you should be comfortable and not notice what you are wearing, and therefore you will be able to focus on the more important things in life.

SELF-ESTEEM WHEN YOU ARE DISABLED— AN INTERVIEW WITH SUE ALCORN

I first met Sue Alcorn in a writer's chat room. Actually, we met when I posted a message about discrimination. She introduced herself and we corresponded, then met in the chat room, and ended up on ICQ (an instant messaging system) together. After a while we exchanged addresses and phone numbers and became good friends.

Sue is a writer, a brilliant woman, and so much fun that I miss her when we don't talk for a few days. She is lovely. Born in Rockville, Connecticut, in 1956, she was raised in New England and settled in New Jersey in 1972. Sue's worked in many fields, including marketing, law, and publishing. In 1992 at the age of 35, she became disabled with a bone disease and to date has survived forty-eight surgeries. She is an advocate for the disabled and is writing a book about her experiences.

Yasmine: How would you describe your attitude toward movement and your own body before you were disabled? Would you have classified yourself as an active, athletic person?

Sue: I was not a very athletic person. Before I became disabled, I enjoyed golfing, swimming, and hiking, but I never participated in a team sport. I'm not a competitive person by nature. During the 1980s, when jogging and exercise became fads, I bought into it for about five minutes by joining an exercise class. But back then, most of my time was spent working. I did a lot of walking, if that counts. I was active in my community and always busy. I managed a hotline for battered women at a shelter, was married, worked ten-hour days, sang in my church choir, went to church every Sunday, helped our women's group with the homeless, and was a Big Sister. So activities-wise, yes, I was always busy. Athletics—hated them!

Yasmine: So many people find themselves nervous asking about disabilities. I sometimes feel that way too, but believe it's better to just come out and ask. What is your disability and how did it change your life on a physical and emotional level?

Sue: My disability wasn't instantaneous. In other words, I wasn't hit by a car or thrown from a motorcycle. My bone disease, avascular necrosis, went misdiagnosed for ten months. AVN affects the joints. Blood doesn't get to the joint area and so the joint dies and collapses.

Apparently the disease was not detectable by any tests in the beginning and kept the doctors guessing and me in excruciating pain. When a woman goes to a doctor complaining of pain, the first thing she is told is "It's all in your head, honey" or "If you just lose a little weight, you'll be fine." I despise that attitude, I find it antiquated and stereotypical. Needless to say, medical technology was not as welcoming or comforting as I'd hoped. There were no doctors who held my hand. They depended on enormous machines spewing out statistics, pictures, and graphs. Marcus Welby was nowhere to be found.

Even when I was properly diagnosed, there were no fast and sure fixer-uppers. There were reconstructive surgeries, prosthetic surgeries, and plastic surgery. With each surgery I was assured that it would get me walking again. Well, fate had another blow for me which complicated my original bone disease: infection. Somehow, somewhere in the myriad of hospitals and rehab centers, I was hit by a super bug, MRSA—methocylin resistant staph aureus. I lost one of my hip replacements to that nasty bug and now only have one hip.

Emotionally it was a roller coaster ride. With each surgery, I hoped I'd get my old life back, but it never happened. I worked hard through all of the rehab and home physical therapy sessions and would walk for a month or two after each surgery, but the disease kept getting worse. After I had one prosthesis put into my right leg, I was able to walk for about six months, but then my left hip wore out.

I think what kept me going during those first years was the hope I'd walk again and be able to go back to work. Once it was clear that this was not going to be an option, I faced some very difficult issues, one of them being my anger. I'm a manic depressive to begin with and it took every fiber of my being to stay on my medication. I wanted the manic phase back, that feeling of euphoria and invincibility. It was what I wanted to cling to most. Luckily, I stayed on my medication and was able to work through my anger with the help of therapists and biofeedback. After the anger abated, I was slowly able to accept my disability.

Yasmine: I can't help but think, since our spirit is tied to our body, that this must have altered in some way how you felt about your spiritual path.

Sue: Good question. I'm happy you asked. I had a profound spiritual experience in 1992 after one of my first major surgeries. The experience changed my view of God and religion, and altered my spiritual path. I was being transported to a rehab center about a half hour away from the hospital and was in excruciating pain. The paramedics loaded me into the back of the ambulance, closed the doors, and we started our journey. I remember one of them sitting behind me asking me questions, while the other one drove. The drone of the questions and the noise of the engine exacerbated my pain, and I remember crying out—deep from within my soul—for the pain, the world, everything to stop.

At that moment, a bright light hovered above me and the face of a woman appeared. I was bathed in warmth—I know this is a cliché, but this is how it happened—and I was swathed in a peace I'd never felt before. The woman was innately familiar to me. I knew her, yet I didn't. She had a smile on her face. I felt a sort of love I'd never felt before and she said to me, "Sue, you'll be okay. Know that you are loved and being watched over and taken care of." And just as fast as she came to me, she left.

I think that was the first time in my life I'd ever experienced what you would call the Divine. I've sat in church pews, read the Bible, listened to sermons, but nothing touched me as strongly as this experience. And I knew at that moment in time that Jesus, Buddha, or Allah are not the only ways to experience God. We are all connected in one way or another to the universal spirit.

Yasmine: I know you experience a great deal of pain in your particular condition. What do you do on a mental/spiritual basis to approach the pain?

Sue: I use a lot of visualization techniques and meditation to help with my pain, in addition to taking regular pain medication. Here's one technique I use with quite a bit of success. When I'm not able to escape the pain and it's just me and the pain, instead of giving in to it, I define it and give it texture and color.

Pain Control Exercise

I do this while lying quietly in my bed, no music, no sound, nothing to distract me. For instance, sometimes pain is difficult to locate—say, for example, a headache. You may have a headache and not realize that the pain really is stemming from behind your left eye or cheek and may be sinus-related rather than tension.

Once I locate the pain, I give it a form—does it feel circular? Is it rough, triangular, oblong, etc.? I concentrate on that for a while, then I give it depth, weight, height, and texture. I watch my breathing and try to take calming breaths as I concentrate on the "object."

Then I give it color—I ask "What color are you?" or "What size are you?" Sometimes it's scarlet, other times it's orange. In some cases there is no color—just blackness. After I've been able to pinpoint it and give it a form, I visualize myself decreasing it. And I keep making it smaller until the pain subsides, which it usually does.

I don't recommend this therapy in place of taking prescribed medication, but I use it for common headaches (instead of taking an aspirin), and in most instances for pain which won't allow me to concentrate on anything else.

Yasmine: What keeps you going? What pushes you through the rough spots?

Sue: Knowing that the rough moment or difficult time is only temporary and, like nature, will change over the course of time. The rough spots for me are life challenges. We were all put here on this Earth, and we each have lessons that must be learned, and we have the free will to ignore those lessons. But it has been my experience that any lesson not learned the first time will crop up later in life and will continue cropping up until that lesson is learned. Spiritually, that's what I'm here on this planet for: to become a better person, and hopefully touch other people along my journey. Laughter is the best medicine, and I was blessed with a great sense of humor. But more important, I think other people, those who are now living and those who have gone before, help me plug along in this life. I learn from their lessons, their triumphs, and their tragedies too.

Yasmine: How has your disability changed you physically, mentally, and spiritually?

Sue: Physically, I'm not able to walk—this is no big deal. I don't think my disability has made me less human, although there are people in this world who don't agree with me. Mentally, because of the extra stress involved, the lithium and Prozac I take had to be increased, but that was to be expected. Where my mental health is concerned, I try to make sure that I follow through with all my appointments. I'm not able to handle spellwork, and this severely hampers my work with energy. Spiritually, I know that there's nothing in the world that I cannot work through. You can't go through forty-eight surgeries in seven years without them affecting your whole person.

My disability has taught me patience. For the first time in my life, I'm comfortable in my own skin—physically and spiritually. Our future is built on the day-to-day choices we make. Perhaps I'm a bit more careful or thoughtful about what I spend my time on than before I became ill. I used to spend a lot of time worrying about the small things in life and also the things I had no control over. Now I find ways to occupy my time by working on my writing, disability advocacy, reading, and a myriad of other activities.

Yasmine: How has this experience affected your sensual and sexual self? How do you cope with the sexual, or non-sexual (as the case usually is) stereotypes that our society pins on disabled persons? What frustrates you? What gives you hope regarding this issue?

Sue: The first question that usually comes up is, "Can you have sex? Does it hurt?" And my response most of the time is "Can *you* have sex and does it hurt?" I suppose people have a lot of questions regarding people with disabilities and their sex lives. It frustrates me that able-bodied people don't educate themselves before asking such questions. Sometimes it's more a morbid curiosity. Of course we have sex. Maybe many positions are not physically possible for us, but we don't lose our sex drive because we have a disability.

My disability has not changed how I view myself sexually. I still wear sexy lingerie and love the way it feels. I may not have a partner at this moment in time, but I think it's important to primp, and I wear satin and lace. My sexual urges are as strong as they have ever been, maybe even stronger. I'm in my forties and currently going through a divorce. There were many years when I was very ill and could not have sex at all. But I am very lucky to have a doctor with whom I can talk openly. And when the time came that I was able to have sex again, he gave me a booklet with a wide variety of sexual positions. He went over them with me, and crossed off the ones that would be bad for my hips and those that I should not do for at least six months.

What gives me hope is with the advent of the ADA[4] many establishments now have made their facilities handicapped accessible. And now that we have more mobility and more access, we are able to interact with the able-bodied world. This aspect promotes more communication between us, and the "mystery" about being disabled is sort of fading away.

Yasmine: How do you cope with exercise and the body's need for movement?

Sue: I can't stress the importance of exercise and movement strongly enough, even if people are bed bound. I was stuck in bed for a good three years with my disability and there were times when the pain was so bad, I couldn't move at all. However, you must move and keep active. If the person is bed bound, make sure he or she is rotated to the side every two hours. Otherwise the skin breaks down and the patient can end up with bedsores. If you are able to move, try flexing your muscles, buttocks, calves, thighs, or arms. Any part of you that moves, move it. If you are not able to move it yourself, have someone do it for you—ask for a massage; everyone loves a good massage.

If you are able to transfer from bed to walker, cane, or wheelchair, try doing bed exercises to start out with. Extend your leg out to the side and return it. Start with repetitions of ten. Repeat with the other leg. Rotate your ankles clockwise and then counterclockwise. However you choose to do your exercises, make sure you do the same number of repetitions on each extremity. For upper body strength, take an old broom handle, lie on your back with the broomstick in both hands and raise it so it's eye level and hold it for a count of three, and lower it back down to your hips. These are simple exercises that you can do yourself if you have been inactive because of your disability.

With any sudden disability, or any disability for that matter, your doctor will most commonly prescribe the amount of activity you are able to do and you'll probably work with a physical therapist (or terrorist, as I so fondly call them). I found that if I did five more repetitions of each prescribed exercise, I got stronger more quickly.

In the beginning, exercise is very painful, but the rewards are wonderful. The more you work at it, the quicker your pain will decrease, more than you could ever imagine. Remember, those muscles and bones have been through a lot and need time to mend, but they also need to keep moving.

If you're not sure what type of exercise(s) you should be doing, check with your doctor before starting any program.

Yasmine: Do you have more or less fear of trying new things, considering what you've experienced? Are changes easier to make now?

Sue: I'm less fearful of trying new things. As I stated previously, surviving forty-eight surgeries does build character in some aspects. I'm not afraid to try anything new. Changes are much easier to assimilate and I welcome them warmly. Sexually, I'm more open-minded than I've ever been.

Yasmine: When you look at yourself now, knowing your future is different than you had planned, what do you foresee?

Sue: As I stated earlier, our future is built on the choices we make today. In my future, I see a lot more challenges medically. I'm writing a book about my experience and hope it will get published one of these days. But for the most part I feel good about the future—no matter what it brings. I want to remain as independent as I can.

Living in a barrier-free apartment complex has opened up a whole new world for me. I have access to transportation now and can do my own shopping, cleaning, cooking, etc. One of these days I'd love to get a van that has hand controls and a lift. I also recently got a power chair, which gives me much more mobility. So, my future is all about being independent and maintaining my independence.

Yasmine: What advice would you give those people who might find themselves in a similar situation? What would you like to tell them about coping with disability and enjoying life to its fullest?

Sue: I think it's important if you are having a hard time dealing with your disability to find someone to talk to. Reach out to any programs available in your town or county. I also think it's important for you to try to be as independent as you can. I don't care if you're hooked up to a respirator and require twenty-four-hour care. You're still human and need time to at least try *something*. People must get out of their comfort zone, disabled or not. So if you are hooked up to a respirator and require twenty-four-hour care, change your routine, read or have someone read you something you are not familiar with. Dare to dream and fantasize. Do something that gets your adrenaline going, take up a new hobby, or go online to the many disabled chat rooms or e-mail groups. There's a whole new world out there on the Internet and there are thousands upon thousands of disabled Web sites. Networking with other disabled and non-disabled people is important. You can keep up with the newest or latest discovery regarding some diseases. There are advocacy groups that could use volunteers. Keep busy, keep interested, and never give up or give in.

Yasmine: What would you like to tell those people who aren't sure of how to react to a friend who suddenly finds himself or herself disabled? What do you wish your friends would have done or not done?

Sue: Excellent question. Friends and family take your disability almost as badly as we ourselves do in the beginning. It's an overwhelming experience for everyone involved. I think the most important thing for friends and family to do at the beginning is let us work through the various issues ourselves. There will be lots of tears, anger, and guilt in the relationship. When you try to do something to help the situation, don't expect your gesture to end the tears or anger. I'm not saying you should abandon your friend or relative. Just know that there are going to be some really rough times we have to go through in order to process our grief.

The biggest issue newly disabled people have to deal with is losing their independence—they will feel as though they are a burden. As hard as it may be for you, don't ever look at the newly disabled with pity. This won't help them or you. You all need to work through it together. I think the most important thing you can do is to make sure they follow the medical plan or advice given by their doctor, help them stick to a good diet, and make sure they are getting the proper sleep and physical therapy. In fact, all parties involved should be taking extra good care of themselves so they can be there to help. You're not going to be of any help if you haven't slept or if you neglect your own personal care.

For those of you who are squeamish, find some way to buck up. This is not happening to you, it's happening to your friend. If you don't think your friend or family member is receiving the proper care or needs help, i.e., if everyone in the family works and there's no one home during the day to help, contact your county or state Social Services agency so that you can find qualified home care to relieve the family. Search the government pages in your telephone book for counseling and daycare programs, for any kind of financial help that your family may need during this difficult time. There are a lot of helpful programs out there. I also suggest you get in touch with a good social worker who can counsel the whole family.

Keep your eye open for depression and address it as soon as possible. It may be temporary and the person may need medication, but there are other things that are important to alleviate the depression. Keep a daily routine going—wake the patient up at a certain time each day, turn on his or her favorite music, read the newspaper, make sure he or she has a good breakfast. Take the person to the mall or grocery store, or ask her or him to run errands if that's possible. Perhaps your friend has favorite TV programs or movies he or she likes to watch. If you can get the person back on the schedule he or she used to be on, this is an enormous help.

Try not to have every friend or relative visit at the same time in the beginning. Make the sessions more one-on-one. Intersperse them throughout the day. Never overload the newly disabled person, unless it's something he or she asks for. Heck, if he or she wants to have a party—have it.

But what is most important to know is that newly disabled people will be exhibiting unusual behavior and that it is only a temporary condition. Remember—they have lost either their ability to walk or some kind of motor activity, and they will feel like a burden. But they are still, and will always be, the people you knew. Don't ever give up on them. I lost a lot of friends due to my disability, but it didn't happen overnight. I used to be quite the social butterfly. But since none of my friend's houses were handicapped accessible, I was unable to go to the dinner parties, barbecues, etc. It's not that expensive to have a ramp built so that your friend can get into your house. I wish my friends had done that for me. Only one did.

Yasmine: Any last thoughts on the subject?

Sue: I think the only thing I'd like to add and emphasize is that the disabled community is really no different from able-bodied people. We may physically look different and may not be able to do all the things an able-bodied person can do, but it's important to get the word out that we are just like anyone else. We laugh, cry, love, hate—we basically feel the same way any human being does. Our IQs don't plunge just because we happen to be sitting instead of standing.

We are sexual creatures and have the same wants and desires able-bodied people do. I've belonged to many disabled e-mail groups where we discuss our favorite sexual positions. It would surprise a lot of "normal" people to know that there are many of us who are into the S&M and B&D scenes. We love leather and lace like anyone else. We are sensual; sometimes we can be downright perverted—just like "normal" people. So, when you're going about your daily routine and happen to see someone in a wheelchair, he or she just might have something sensual going on underneath his or her clothes or might have had the wildest sex ever imagined the night before! You never know!

Yasmine: Thank you for giving me this interview, Sue. I know through our talks I've come to learn much about your world and the way the world in general perceives you. I only wish that people who can see so clearly on some issues weren't so blind on this one.

---

1. See chapter 4.
2. See *Sexual Ecstasy and the Divine*.
3. Diaphragm: a muscular membranous partition separating the abdominal and thoracic cavities and functioning in respiration. When you breathe from the diaphragm, your breath will be deeper and your lower abdomen should expand.
4. The ADA is the American Disability Act. Signed by President George Bush in July 1990, this is the first comprehensive civil rights bill for Americans with disabilities and was a landmark moment.

CHAPTER FOUR

Bathing and Beauty Rituals

Blessed be Oh Lady of the Waters
May I swim forever within thy embrace.

—Diane MarieChild, "Earth Songs"

Water makes up between fifty-five and seventy-five percent of the average human body and between seventy-five and eighty-five percent of the human brain. We are of the ocean. On an almost molecular level, we are connected to the same force the moon extends to the tides, their ebb and flow. We are filled with fluids: blood, tears, sweat, urine, amniotic liquid if we're pregnant, mucus, semen, phlegm, and so much more. I caught you grimacing—sounds messy, doesn't it?

Well, yes, it is messy. Messy and sticky and not at all neat and packaged the way the media tends to portray our bodies. But you know, life *is* sticky and dirty and wet. Deal with it.

At the same time, water cleanses us, runs through us, clears our systems, cleans our skin. The sound of raindrops falling or waves lapping soothes our minds. Water is one of the four major Elements called upon in our rituals. It serves as a symbol for the subconscious, for emotions, and the hidden depths of the psyche. Ritual baths have long been used to purify and cleanse the self. Water empowers our magickal practice.

The chalice, symbol of the Element of Water, is used during the Hieros Gamos.

Ritual bathing is the perfect medium for spellcraft for beauty magick. What better way to increase glamour and natural attributes than to use a ritual bath.

THE RITUAL BATH

Immersion in sacred or charged waters has long been a method of both purification and rebirth. Baptism can be linked to this practice, as can the Jewish Mikvah rituals. When you approach the ritual bath, you should do so with reverence. The ritual bath can be used for many purposes, and here I present an outline that can be tailored to your individual needs and tastes.

Always approach the bath with already-clean skin. Take a quick shower to wash away the grime and sweat of the day. If you want to shave your legs or underarms, do so during this time.

Coordinate the candles, incense, and music to fit the type of ritual you are performing. Bear in mind that a stick of incense in a large room may be perfect, but in a small and enclosed space it may be overwhelming. You might wish to burn a little of it before you begin the ritual and then snuff it out so the scent lingers but does not choke you. Or you may wish to forego incense and use potpourri instead.

On pages 78-79 you will find a table of correspondences to help you plan your ritual.

If you conduct your ritual bath in a bathroom, as opposed to a natural water source (see the following section), try to clean the area first. If your room is neat and tidy, the magick won't be fraught with chaos, and you will be more comfortable. Try to ensure privacy as you would with any ritual, and remember, *never* allow an electrical appliance, such as a cassette deck, too near the tub. You don't want your ritual bath to become your last rite.

You may wish to cast a Circle, or you may choose to forego this step. If you decide to cast a Circle, do so when you've assembled everything you need. Light your candles, cast your Circle, and call the Element of Water:

Oh Spirit of the Water,
I call to thee from the heart of my heart,
You who are the Undines of the raging Rivers,
You who are the Naiads of the still Grottos and
The Sirens of the crashing ocean breakers.
Come to me, Spirit of the Oceans,
You who are the tears of our bodies,
You who guard the hidden depths of our psyches.
Come to this Circle and join my rites,
Bring your energy and purify me, strengthen my magick
And lead me into your realm.

After you have invoked the Spirit of Water, fill your tub, using the appropriate bath salts, oils, herbs, or bubble bath for your ritual. When you step into the tub, visualize stepping into that energy, into a lake of beauty, or prosperity, or purification—whatever you are focusing on in your ritual.

As you lean back in the tub, let your mind drift and feel the water's connection to your skin. Feel the gentle movement of the waves as you shift your body. After a few moments, focus your attention. Spend about twenty minutes visualizing the results you want from your ritual. Feel the energy of the oils and candles and incense, of the water itself, working for and with you. Slowly let yourself sink more and more into the visualization and begin to chant the affirmation that goes with your particular rite. Build the power. If you want, you can splash the water in rhythm to it, or you can use the energy of sex through masturbation to build the energy.[1] When the power peaks, release it to your goal. Gently allow yourself to relax again. Then, when you are ready leave the tub, take a quick shower if you like, and open your Circle.

VARIOUS RITUAL BATHS AND THEIR CORRESPONDING ENERGIES

Ritual	Candle Colors	Bath Salts	Runes[2]
Beauty	Rose	Rose	Lagaz
	Pink	Honeysuckle	Kenaz
	Teal	Peach	Berkana
Lust/Sex	Red	Jasmine	Neid
	Gold	Ylang ylang	Gebo
	Beeswax	Vanilla	
Love	Red	Rose	Neid
	Green	Orange blossom	Gebo
	Pink	Vanilla	Wunjo
Movement/Exercise	Green	Spice	Sigel
	Gold	Orange blossom	Uruz
	Brown	Spring rain	Kenaz
Prosperity	Green	Honeysuckle	Fehu
	Gold	Patchouli	Othel
	Brown	Jasmine	Jera
Purification	White	Lavender	Tir
	Silver	Lemon	Siegel
	Lavender	Peppermint	
Psychic Powers	Purple	Honeysuckle	Eihwaz
	Indigo	Citron	Perdhro
	Silver	Rose	Ansuz
Intellect	Yellow	Lily of the valley	Ansuz
	White	Peach	Mannaz
			Lagaz
Protection	White	Violet	Algiz
	Gold	Primrose	Berkana
	Hyacinth		Raido

Ritual	Flowers	Herbs[3]	Affirmations
Beauty	Roses Orange blossom	Witch hazel Heather Thyme	My inner and outer beauty radiate and shine.
Lust/Sex	Roses Violets Jasmine	Cardamom Parsley Lemongrass	I magnetize passion into my life and feel the full joy of my sexual nature.
Love	Roses Orange blossom Geranium	Rosemary Spearmint Vervain	Love enters my life and I am open to both giving and receiving it in a healthy manner.
Movement/Exercise	Fern Larkspur Life-everlasting	Marjoram Nutmeg Thyme	I experience health and movement and embrace the active nature of my body.
Prosperity	Trillium Tulip Honesty	Basil Patchouli Chamomile	Prosperity fills my life and abundance surrounds my days.
Purification	Lavender Iris Rosemary	Chamomile Fennel Vervain	I release that which is no longer necessary in my life and let go of stagnation.
Psychic Powers	Honeysuckle Rose Yarrow	Lemongrass Mugwort Uva ursi	My psychic self opens to the Divine and I accept and revel in my abilities.
Intellect	Wisteria Lily of the valley	Rosemary Sage Eyebright	I am wise, learn quickly, and remember what I observe and hear.
Protection	Cactus African violet Carnation	Mint Wintergreen Witch hazel	I cloak myself in a robe of protection and strengthen my boundaries.

Outdoor Ritual Bathing

Performing a ritual bath outdoors requires that you find a natural grotto, lake, stream, or beach where you can shed your clothes and have the privacy you need. It has always been my belief and practice when I'm outside performing ritual in the heart of nature to use few tools or props, and instead to let the energy of the wild work its magick on me.

You will perhaps want only a candle or two (in a glass holder that won't tip and that is protected from the wind, so you don't risk a fire or having your light go out), a towel and robe, and a simple meal to eat afterward in the cradle of the forest or beach.

It is also a good idea to go with a friend who can keep watch. There are unfortunately all sorts of psychos and wackos loose in the world today, and if one should stumble upon you (whether you're male or female) while you are nude in the woods, you might find yourself in trouble, so use your common sense. Make sure your friend can swim. You never know what might happen in a Circle or in a strange body of water. Even the strongest swimmer may get disoriented for a myriad of reasons.

When you approach the body of water you've designated for your ritual bath, you will want to feel the energy of the area. Ask permission from the spirits of the land and water to hold a magickal rite and truly be honest about what reaction you get. When you are given the go-ahead, find a safe space to set out your candles. Cast your Circle in the same way you would if you were indoors, but focus on the variants of energy you would not always find in an enclosed human-made space.

Call the Elements. When you are working outdoors, it pays to call all four Elements rather than just the Spirit of Water. You will want the guidance and help of all that is around you.

Do not take soap or bath salts into the lake or ocean; you do not want to pollute the environment. Instead, after your invocation of the Elements and deities (should you wish to work with the gods), invoke the spirit of that energy which you seek, i.e., prosperity, love, lust, beauty. Ask the spirit of that energy to bless you and to bless the waters in which you bathe and to charge you with energy so that you might manifest it in your life.

Then, with your friend keeping watch, remove your clothes and slide into the water. Once you are in the water, adjust to the temperature, then slowly connect with the spirit of the lake, grotto, etc., and let the energy flow through you, cleansing you, charging you. Visualize your goal, see it grow and manifest, feel the energy of the water swell around you, bathing you in magickal light.

When you begin chanting, start to cone the energy and then peak it, releasing it to go out into the universe and manifest. Relax, emerge from the water, towel dry, and eat a small but nourishing meal to renew your strength.

Witch Hazel-Rose Water Toner

When you are going out for a special evening, before you apply your makeup, you might want to rinse your face with witch hazel–rose water. Not only is it a good astringent, it also contains the magickal energies of beauty and bewitchment.

To prepare a batch (and you will want to make small batches and keep them refrigerated between uses), pour one quart of bottled spring water into a non-metallic saucepan. Bring to a slow boil and remove it from the heat. Add a muslin bag containing one cup of witch hazel and one cup of rose petals. Cover and steep for thirty minutes. Remove the herbs and, if necessary, strain the liquid into a clean and sterilized bottle.

Cork and store in the refrigerator. After washing your face, apply it liberally with cotton balls, especially under your eyes and around your chin and nose. Allow your skin to air dry. You may use this on other areas of your body that are in need of toning too, such as the breasts or the hands.

Lemon Cleansing Ritual

When we make the decision to eat better, to start exercising, and to get more sleep, we inevitably come to a place where we want to detoxify our bodies. It helps if we perform a ritual to jump-start our resolve, as well as to set the mood for the days to come.

On the night before you begin your new regime, prepare the following: Bring sixteen ounces of bottled water (like Perrier) to just below boiling. Add two tablespoons of honey. When the honey has dissolved, remove the pot from the heat and add the juice of two lemons and one mint teabag. Cool the pot, remove the teabag, and pour the drink into a glass jar into which you have placed a thoroughly scrubbed clear quartz crystal.

Set the jar in the sunlight for two hours to absorb the healing rays of the sun, then remove the crystal and drink the liquid while focusing on strengthening your will power, your desire to change to better habits, and how much you love yourself in order to make this effort.

Mielikki's Beauty Spell

I developed this spell to use in conjunction with my Goddess, who is, among other things, a goddess of the Hunt and of Faerie. Steeped in faerie magick, it is designed to invite the energy of the Fey into your life to charm your spirit and your beauty.

Twice each month, under the Full and New Moons, set an altar with these things: a purple (plum) candle in a brass or crystal holder; an image of a bee, a stag or reindeer, and a bear; a representation of the Koad Ogham rune; a pentacle or pentagram; flowers, preferably foxglove, wildflowers, or deep red roses; a chalice of mead, cranberry vodka, or cranberry juice if you do not drink alcohol. The cloth should be green or purple or a combination of both colors. Let no iron touch the altar. There should be a mirror near the altar in which you can look at yourself. Light a stick of honeysuckle or violet incense.

You may add these things to the altar if you wish: antlers; crystal figurines of unicorns, stags, bears, bees; fur, preferably bear or wolf; a decorative bottle of honey; moonstone, peridot, and garnet beads and stones.

Have music ready to play, preferably Gabrielle Roth or Dead Can Dance, or a CD like *Eternal Egypt* by Phil Thornton and Hossam Ramzy.

Cast a Circle, beginning in the North, and then invoke the Elements in this manner. Turn toward the North and say:

Spirits of the Earth,
Spirit of Maa
You who are stone and rock, bone, and crystal,
You who are tree and root and branch,
You, whose soil is the body of the Goddess
And whose grass is the green of Her hair,
Spirit of Earth, come to me!
Spirit of the Wolf, Spirit of the Para,
I call upon thee.
You who rule from the blackest caverns below
To the highest mountaintops,
Hear me.
Bring to these rites your spirit of materialization,
Of strength and manifestation.

Begin to turn deosil (clockwise), focusing a line of Earth energy through your hand or athame. Make one full sweep, saying:

With a ring of stone and bone and crystal,
I encircle this sacred space and all within.
Let nothing enter unwelcome.

Draw an invoking pentacle in the air, facing the North, and say:

Spirit of the Earth, welcome and blessed be!

Now, turn and face the East. Raise your hand or athame and say:

Spirits of the Air,
Spirit of Ilma,
You who are mist and vapor and cloud,
You who are fresh breeze and wild hurricane,
You who weave the Web at the edge of Dawn
Sweeping out stagnation to weave the new day,
Come to me.
Spirit of the Hawk, Spirit of the Terhi,
Hear me.
Bring into these rites purification,
Sweep through and remove stagnation
And allow me to grow and radiate in clarity.

Begin to turn deosil, focusing a line of Air energy through your hand or athame. Make one full circle, saying:

With a ring of mist and vapor and fog
I encircle this sacred space and all within
Let nothing enter unwelcome.

Draw an invoking pentacle in the air, facing the East, and say:

Spirit of the Air, welcome and blessed be!

Turn and face the South. Raise your hand or athame into the air and say:

Spirit of the Flame,
Spirit of Tuli,
You who are the crackle of bonfires
You who are the golden sun and glowing lava,
You who are the heat of the desert, and the
Sparkle of phosphorescence on the shore and
In the water,
Come to me.
Spirit of the Phoenix,
Spirit of Etelätär
Hear me.
Bring into these rites your spirit of passion,
Your fearsome beauty and
Ability to transmute and rise new from the
Ashes.

Begin to turn deosil, focusing a line of Fire energy through your hand or athame. Make one full circle, saying:

With a ring of sunlight and lava, I encircle this
Sacred space and all within
Let nothing enter unwelcome.

Draw an invoking pentacle in the air, facing the South, and say:

Spirit of the Flame, welcome and blessed be!

Turn and face the West. Raise your hand or athame into the air and say:

Spirit of Vesi,
You who are the Moon Mother,
You who are the Undines of the Rivers
And the Sirens of the crashing ocean breakers
You who are the Naiads of the Grottos,
Come to me.
Spirit of the Water,
Spirit of the Shark,
Hear me.
Bring to these rites your deepest intuition
And truest emotions,
Teach me to be flexible, to adapt and flow
Like your waters.

Begin to turn deosil, focusing a line of Water energy through your hand or athame. Make one full circle, saying:

With a ring of wave and rain and tears
I encircle this sacred space and all within
Let nothing enter unwelcome.

Draw an invoking pentacle in the air, facing the West, and say:

Spirit of the Water, welcome and blessed be!

Light the candle, and invoke Mielikki:

Mielikki, Queen of Fey
Enchantress of the Silver Forest
Green-clothed in gossamer silk

Spun by dreaming spiders,
You who are Dark Huntress
Creeping through treetops
With your poison-tipped arrows,
Hear me.
You who wear the antlered crest,
Come to me.

Mielikki, Mistress of Tapiola,
You are the emerald forest in
The glimmering sunlight of afternoon
And the sparkling phosphorescence
That glistens on the beach at midnight.
Starlight Stag Mother, Mother Bear,
Queen of Bees,
The branches of Your forest
Drip with golden honey
And silver chimes sing out Your
Name on the wind.

Mielikki, Protectress of animals,
Join my rite, open the Gate
To Your Crystal Grove,
Bathe me in golden-green flames
And let me quench my thirst
From Your sparkling sapphire pool.
Lady of Tapiola, welcome, and Blessed Be!

Drink a toast to Mielikki, then look into the mirror and repeat the following. If you can't memorize it, at least read through it several times to get the feel for the flow of the words. As you chant, feel the words sinking into your being, feel the energies responding to your call.

I call upon my inner strength
Earth, Air, Fire, Water,
I call upon Mielikki,
The forest's sylvan daughter.
Powers of Faerie come to me,
Undines, sirens of the sea.
Let me sing my Siren Song,
Let its reach be loud and long.
Let me breathe the fire that burns
Green amongst the forest's ferns.
Let me sparkle like shore and sea,
Phosphorescence shines in me.
I radiate compelling charm.
Strength from deepest cavern's walls
Flows through my legs and arms.
Windswept peak of ice and snow
Clears my mind and lets it soar.
Lake and river, pool and streams,
Clarify my moods and dreams.

Beauty gleams from my [long and] radiant hair.
Beauty shines from my eyes.
Beauty radiates from my smile.
Beauty graces my confident shoulders.
Beauty floats from the touch of my hands.
Beauty crests from my milk-white [alter to suit coloring] bosom.
Beauty curves around my soft, gentle belly.

Beauty supports my strong buttocks.
Beauty supports my woman's thighs.
Beauty strengthens my calves and ankles.
Beauty dances from my feet.

Now, turn on the music and dance for at least ten minutes. Let yourself flow into the rhythm, feel it moving through you. Express the music, become the music, and know you are beautiful.

You may use this as a basis for creating rituals with other goddesses, but I ask that you please do not alter the invocation to Mielikki; I wrote that especially for my Lady, as her Priestess. Write something new instead. For other beauty spells, you might want to refer to my book, *Embracing the Moon.*[4]

---

1. See *Sexual Ecstasy and the Divine.*
2. Carve runes on the candles or on the bar of soap you are using.
3. Fill a muslin bag with these herbs and steep in two cups boiling water for ten minutes. Add to bath water.
4. See *Embracing the Moon* by Yasmine Galenorn, Llewellyn Publications, 1998.

CHAPTER FIVE

The Divine Nature of Beauty

Behold the chariot of the Fairy Queen!
Celestial coursers paw the unyielding air;
Their filmy pennons at her word they furl,
And stop obedient to the reins of light;
These the Queen of Spells drew in;
She spread a charm around the spot,
And, leaning graceful from the ethereal car,
Long did she gaze, and silently,
Upon the slumbering maid.

—Percy Bysshe Shelley, "Queen Mab"

Once Aphrodite stepped from the ocean, mankind would never be the same. The foam-born goddess of beauty could outshine the sun, and we fell at her feet, captives of her heart. Throughout the ages there have been deities of grace from all cultures, in all shapes, sizes, and colors. And each one possessed a unique and exquisite beauty. Below is a brief listing of some of the goddesses and gods of beauty, a little about their background, and correspondences if known. Where correspondences are difficult to find, I've made suggestions (noted by an asterisk).

THE DIVINE NATURE OF BEAUTY

Deity and Origin	Description	Corresponding Energies
Adonis: Greek God	Originally thought to descend from Tammuz and Dumuzi, Adonis is a god of rebirth, of vegetation, and renewal. He is also connected with incredible physical beauty and love.	Gems: peridot, diamond, topaz Flowers: narcissus, vine, laurel Animals: lion, phoenix Perfumes: narcissus, jasmine
Apollo: Greek God	Lord of the sun, music, and poetry, he took control of the Muses and the Oracle of Delphi. Brilliant and shining, he epitomized male form and symmetry.	Gems: jacinth, topaz, diamond Flowers: sunflower, heliotrope Animals: crab, sphinx, centaur Perfumes: amber, lotus
Aphrodite: Greek Goddess	Foam-born of the sea, Aphrodite rules over all aspects of love, sexuality, and beauty. She is married to Hephaestus, ugly god of the forge, showing the attraction of opposites, and often has dalliances with Ares, where we see the connection of love and hate.	Gems: emerald, turquoise Flowers: rose, clover, myrtle Animals: dove, swan, sparrow Perfumes: rose, red sandalwood
Arianrhod: Welsh Goddess	Goddess of the stars, Arianrhod rules over the Caer Arianrhod in the skies. She is a goddess of reincarnation, shadow-work, and beauty.	*Gems: diamond, silver *Flowers: white rose, lily Animals: sow, owl *Perfumes: gum mastic, jasmine
Balder: Norse God	God of the sun, lord of beauty and happiness, Balder was killed by Loki but will return from the dead after Ragnarok to help re-create the race of the gods.	*Gems: carnelian, citrine, amber *Flowers: sunflower, mistletoe *Animals: lion *Perfumes: amber, sandalwood
Bast: Egyptian Goddess	Goddess of cats, the dance, ecstasy, and beauty, Lady Bast is often depicted as lion- or cat-headed. Her rites often included orgiastic ceremonies.	*Gems: peridot, gold, turquoise *Flowers: rose, lotus, fern Animals: cats of all kinds *Perfumes: lotus, orange, amber
Bes: Egyptian God	A dwarf clad in leopard skins with an oversized head, Bes is, among other things, protector of the dead, protector against demons and dangerous animals. He rules over luck, marriage, dance, childbirth, cosmetics, and feminine accessories/jewelry.	*Gems: turquoise, gold *Flowers: lily, lotus *Animals: leopard *Perfumes: amber, lotus

Deity and Origin	Description	Corresponding Energies
Freyja: Norse Goddess	Norse goddess of beauty, sexuality, and war, she is by some accounts married to Odin, by others to another deity. Queen of the Valkyries, she has first pick over those slain in battle. She wears the sacred necklace Brisingamen.	Gems: amber, copper, turquoise Flowers: poppy, rose, cypress Animals: housecat, boar Perfumes: amber, myrrh
Freyr: Norse God	Norse god of the Vanir, brother to Freyja, lord of fertility, sensuality, abundance, joy, and beauty, among other things.	★Gems: amber, copper ★Flowers: rose, cypress Animals: boar ★Perfumes: musk, patchouli
Hathor: Egyptian Goddess	Goddess of pleasure, love, beauty, and competent career women, Hathor supervises over the spheres of cosmetics, adornment, poise, grace, and elegance.	Gems: emerald, turquoise Flowers: rose, myrtle, clover Animals: cow, lion, lynx Perfumes: rose, sandalwood
Inanna: Sumerian Goddess	Queen of Heaven, Inanna rules over love, beauty, battle, magick, weaving, and wine. She is connected with Ishtar and Isis, and is also connected with the Hieros Gamos.	Gems: diamond, pearl, sapphire Flowers: poppy, cypress, lily Animals: lion, snake, scorpion Perfumes: myrrh, musk, narcissus
Ishtar: Assyro-Babylonian Goddess	Goddess of the moon, love, battle, storm, and marriage. She is connected with Inanna and Isis, and is also connected with the Hieros Gamos.	Gems: diamond, sapphire, ruby Flowers: olive, lily, lotus ★Animals: lion, scorpion Perfumes: myrrh, dragon's blood
Isis: Egyptian Goddess	Great Mother of Egypt, Isis is perhaps the best culmination of the concept of the Great Goddess in the world. Married to Osiris, the pair epitomizes the male/female link in nature, and together rule over the land with an unwavering power. Isis is goddess of life and of love, of beauty, fidelity, strength, and magick.	Gems: peridot, sapphire, beryl Flowers: olive, lotus, poppy Animals: sphinx, snake, lion, owl Perfumes: myrrh, musk, narcissus
Lakshmi: Hindu Goddess	The personification of beauty, Lakshmi rules over good fortune and abundance. She forms a triad with Sarasvati and Devi.	Gems: quartz Flowers: willow, lily, ivy Animals: sphinx Perfumes: dittany of Crete
Nuada: Irish God	An Irish king of the Tuatha De Danann, he lost his hand in battle. Since the Celtic kings were required to be physically perfect, he was forced from his throne but regained it when a silver hand was made for him.	★Gems: silver, sapphire ★Flowers: iris, shamrock ★Animals: lion, eagle ★Perfumes: patchouli, vetiver

Deity and Origin	Description	Corresponding Energies
Oshun: Yoruba Goddess	A river goddess, Oshun rules over beauty, love, sex, and childbirth.	Gems: gold, shells, pearl *Flowers: tiger lily, narcissus Animals: peacock, quail, parrot Perfumes: cinnamon, orange
Rauni: Finnish Goddess	Rauni, also known as Akka, rules over grain, the harvest, sexuality, fire, and lightning. She also is connected to the realm of beauty.	*Gems: garnet, citrine, ruby Flowers: rowan *Animals: snake, lizard *Perfumes: orange, cinnamon
Venus: Roman Goddess	Venus is almost interchangeable with Aphrodite at this point, but originally she was also a goddess of spring and vegetation.	Gems: topaz, emerald, turquoise Flowers: rose, myrtle, sunflower Animals: lynx, sparrow, bull, lion Perfumes: red sandalwood, rose
White Tara: Hindu/Tibetan Goddess	Star goddess and teacher of the gods, Tara is connected with Dolma. She rides on a lion, holds the sun in her hands, and is the mother of Buddha, the founder of the lunar dynasties. She is considered the shakti, or female partner, of the Bodhisattva Avalokitesvara.	*Gems: diamond, ruby Flowers: lotus Animals: lion *Perfumes: sandalwood, lotus

If you choose to invoke these deities for ritual, please research them first to make sure that they are the ones you truly want to invoke. Some deities have more than one side; some have dark natures, and you don't want to open up an energy you aren't sure about.

The awe of beauty will always be with us, whether seen in the shape of a Rubenesque woman or a Cindy Crawford type.

GUIDED MEDITATION FOR SELF-ESTEEM

As with all guided meditations, make sure that you properly ground and center yourself before proceeding. Always include the last paragraph in the meditation, and try to eat a bite afterward, preferably protein and some fruit. You may want to tape record this meditation or, if in a group, designate one person to read while the others follow the journey. When you come to a *pause*, allow a thirty-second beat. *Extended pauses* will indicate the time frame on an individual basis.

Relax, get comfortable, and close your eyes. Take three slow, deep breaths and slowly exhale. (*pause*)

You find yourself standing in a large bedroom. Take some time to look around. It is the room of your dreams, with the furniture, drapes, and paintings that you've always imagined owning. You also find a stereo there, and you may put on any music you like which suits your mood. (*extended pause—one minute*)

As the music fills the room, allow it to flow through your body. Focus on the feelings in your body. It is time to get to know and love this temple of flesh within which your spirit resides. (*pause*)

Imagine the following. Start by sitting down on the bed or on the floor or on a chair. Examine your feet. Look at your toes; wiggle them. Run your fingers over your ankles and the tops of your feet. Caress your arches. Don't focus on the problem spots, simply acknowledge them and let the thought go. What do you like about your feet? Think of all they do for you, think of what they mean to you. (*extended pause— one minute*)

Run your hands up your calves. How do they curve? Are they muscled? Straight rather than curved? Do you have any markings on them? If you are a woman, do you shave your legs or not? If you're a man, how hairy are they? Run your hands along your calves and feel the skin glide under your fingers. Enjoy the sensation of touching your calves. What do they do for you? (*extended pause—one minute*)

Now you come to your thighs. What are they like? If you are a woman, do you berate yourself for having hips? Put that thought aside and let your hands glide over your hips, feeling the curves, the skin, the strength in your thighs. Imagine what your thighs can do for you, the power that resides within them. (*extended pause—one minute*)

Run your hands between your legs, up to where your genitals reside. If you are a man, take hold of your cock. Feel how it rests in your hand, the difference between when it's flaccid and erect. How do you feel about your penis? What does it look like? Are you circumcised or not? How do you feel about that? Now cup your balls in your hand and feel the weight as they rest there. Do they hang evenly or not? Gently examine them.

If you are a woman, slip your fingers between your legs and run them along your vulva. Feel the lips that enfold your urethral opening, clitoris, and vagina. Gently run your fingers over your clitoris. Is it large, small? Notice the sensations you produce when you touch it. How do you feel about your clitoris? Now slide your fingers back and into your vagina. Is it moist? Dry? Are you tense? If so, will your body to relax. If you are a virgin, you will probably still have a hymen, a membrane that covers part of the vagina. However, the hymen can be broken by vigorous exercise as well as through sexual contact. If you still have your hymen, be gentle and note how the membrane feels against your fingers. How do you feel about your vagina? Take some time to make friends with your genitalia. (*extended pause—two minutes*)

Now, bring your hands up to your stomach. If you are like some people, you might find yourself uncomfortable doing this, but try not to judge yourself. Just let your fingers glide across your skin, admire the curve of your belly; if it's flat, feel the smooth stretch of flesh that makes up your abdomen. Try to detach yourself from the negative views you may hold or have held about your stomach in the past. Think about what your abdomen does for you; how your stomach processes the nutrients to keep you alive; how your pancreas and liver and other internal organs work to keep you functioning smoothly. If you're a woman, think about your womb and the monthly cycles that it runs through or has run through in the past. (*extended pause—one minute*)

Bring your hands up to your breasts and chest area. Run your fingers across your nipples and watch how they react. What do they do for your self-image? If you are a mother, perhaps they are a symbol of life-giving milk; if you are childfree, perhaps they are a symbol of your womanhood. If you have been through breast cancer, you may have shame or painful memories attached to this area of your body and it may take some time to work through that. Even if your breasts have been altered through surgery, they are still part of you, still part of your being, and you can reclaim yourself. For a man, your chest might symbolize strength or masculinity. Take a few moments to examine how you relate to your breasts and chest area. (*extended pause—one minute*)

Feel your throat, run your fingers along your face and over your head. Everyone's face is unique; your features, your hair, are yours alone. Feel the bow of your lips, the curve of your nose. Do you have high cheekbones or low ones? How long is your hair, or do you have hair at all? Are your eyebrows bushy or barely there? Treat your face as if your fingers were feeling it for the first time. If you have wrinkles, are they laugh lines? Gently glide your fingers over your skin, getting to know the hollows and curves of your face. (*extended pause—one minute*)

Lastly, take a good look at your hands and your arms. These are the limbs through which you reach out to the world, which allow you to touch others and manipulate your environment. Wiggle your fingers, take a close look at them. What are your nails like: claws, or short and neat? Are your knuckles bony or plump? Are your fingers short and stubby, or are they long and slender? Feel the muscles of your arms—are they taut or soft? What do your hands do for you? Think about all that you accomplish because you have use of these limbs. Spend some time acquainting yourself with your hands and arms. (*extended pause—one minute*)

Now take three deep breaths. You have reconnected with your body and hopefully you've reclaimed some of your beauty and strength. Try to spend some time with your body every day. Get comfortable touching yourself, in intimate places as well as in less private areas. Get to know your body, the arc of your curves, the feel of your own touch.

Let yourself come to rest. Follow my voice. Ten...nine...you are slowly pulling out of trance. Eight...seven...six...you are becoming awake and aware. Five...four...you feel your thoughts quickening and stirring. Three...two...take three deep breaths and when you awaken, you will be refreshed and alert. One...now take another deep breath and open your eyes when you are ready.

Suggested Exercises for Self-Esteem Meditation

- Try the elements of this meditation mentally. After you are comfortable with imagining touching your body, then try it on a physical level.
- If you are uncomfortable with your lover touching you, but your lover says she or he loves your body, perhaps you might want to let him or her help you with this exercise. Realize how much you mean to your lover and how much she or he enjoys your body.
- Take long baths and use perfume, lotion, and powder as a means of touching yourself without feeling too awkward.
- Find something to like about your body every day. Look at yourself in the mirror as you tell yourself what that something is.
- If people make unkind remarks about your body, remember that these remarks probably extend from their own insecurity. If you think it's outright cruelty, stand up for yourself and tell them you will not permit their behavior, and cease talking with them until

they apologize. You don't need people in your life who are going to tear down your self-esteem.

- Remember, there will always be days when you are uncomfortable with your body, and areas of your body that you may not easily find lovable. The key is to find something good about that area without lying to yourself. If you truly have a hard time loving your stomach, try to find one good thing about it. Emphasize that, but figure out realistically what you can do to be more comfortable in your own skin.

Part II

〜

MOVEMENT
AS RITUAL

We were all born to move, to surrender to the beat.
Your soul is a dancer. No effort. No judgment.
Pure energy in the moment.

—Gabrielle Roth, "Frontispiece to Endless Wave"

CHAPTER SIX

The Dream of the Dance

O body swayed to music, O brightening glance
How can we know the dancer from the dance?
            —W.B. Yeats, "Among School Children"

I Am the Swirl of Skirts Dancing
Spikes on polished tile
Hair weaves a nimbus around shoulders
Convolutions in color
I am the swirl of skirts dancing
I am the dream of the divine
Teach me to desire, Mother Song
Set my feet free, Father Drum.
Patterns etched in the wave of a note
Tempo beats the rhythm of blood
Let loose the mind and follow body
Heels tattoo rhythms on spotlit stage
Eyes flash with diamond dreams
Leap into the air, spinning top
I am the swirl of skirts dancing
I am the dream of the divine
Teach me to soar, Mother Song
Set my hunger free, Father Drum.
Vibrations zigzag a metered vision

Cadence beats the coursing of pulse
Let loose the mind and follow body
Anklets jingle against peeling soil
Arms snake in sinuous delight
Flashing hips under veils
I am the swirl of skirts dancing
I am the dream of the divine
Teach me to coil, Mother Song
Set my prayers free, Father Drum.
Echoes rebound off canyon walls
Rhythm beats the pulsing of the heart
Let loose the mind and follow body

—Yasmine Galenorn

Exercise? Who, me? Let's face it, there are those people who are happy campers when they are at their aerobics classes or when they're bopping around the gym in spandex, but most people I know aren't. I love dancing, love wandering in the woods, but I'm basically exercise-challenged. It's hard to carve out the exercise habit. Once I get into it I love it, but I still have a hard time not self-destructing.

Over the years I've noticed that I have a tendency, along with a few other writers I know, to feel I have to focus on either my mind or my body. Sometimes it's hard to find the middle ground and balance both body and spirit, but that's what this book is all about. And so, even as I help you make your own journey, I hope to help myself follow the quest, the flickering flame, the dance of passion.

WHY YOU NEED TO EXERCISE

Movement is vital for the body. Even if you have limited mobility, it's absolutely imperative that you exercise in whatever way you can. Strength keeps you healthy. Muscle may weigh more than fat, but exercise speeds up your metabolism, increases your endurance, and puts a sparkle in your eye that no drug or intoxicant can imitate.

Regular exercise will provide more positive side effects in your life than you thought possible. Besides increasing your sex drive, it will keep you healthier, make you more comfortable in your body, allow you to move with more ease, increase your confidence, make your clothes fit better, and possibly improve your sleep. Regular exercise contributes to heightened muscle tone, which in turn can assist in strengthening your cardiac and respiratory systems and circulation. Blood pressure often drops, since working out releases stresses in a way few other methods do.

There is another side to exercise that is seldom mentioned in instructional tapes and books, but it's one that regular exercisers tend to know about and understand. Often called *the zone,* it's a space you move into the more intense the exercise becomes. I believe it can be found in pursuits such as yoga as well as strenuous dance, running, and aerobics. I also found it when I lifted weights.

Much like a pain threshold, you reach a barrier of discomfort and fatigue during exercise. If you stop right there, you don't push through your limits. You remain at a plateau for long periods of time. But if you can achieve a certain mind set, a frame of thought that allows you to go beyond that pain, to work it through your body and release it, you achieve an altered state of consciousness. The times I've reached this level, it's been like a doorway opened up, like I was suddenly flying. I was then able to break the previous limits on what I could do. During the days when I frequented Pagan festivals, and more privately, I would dance all night around the bonfire. Each time I reached a point where

I became the dance, where I became the energy of the movement and touched the Divine through my body.

Often this state corresponds with the release of endorphins triggered by exercise. Endorphins are a group of morphine-like chemicals which are produced by the brain. Found in spinal fluid and the endocrine system, they are believed to regulate pain receptors and may have some effect on memory, learning, and sex drive. Endorphins create a natural high—remember the term *runner's high?*—and our bodies experience what I consider to be a nonsexual form of orgasm, one that can be just as fulfilling. The achievement of this "zone" requires some meditation and forethought, but it's well worth it.

Visualization for Body Movement

For this exercise I want you to get into a comfortable position, relax, close your eyes, and take three deep breaths. See yourself, as you are, but moving, dancing—participating in whatever form of physical activity you think you would enjoy and feel comfortable doing. What is it you are doing? Watch your body move, and think about the different motions that it goes through. Are you playing alone or with others? Do you think you would be comfortable in a group activity or do you prefer to take more of an individual approach? Take some time to get used to seeing yourself in motion.

See yourself successfully accomplishing a workout. Don't use this visualization to force yourself into the image of a champion gymnast or a world-class bodybuilder. Simply make this a stepping stone to a workout—a motivational image, so to speak. This can be an integral part to success; professional athletes use visualization all the time to increase their abilities and to motivate themselves. Try to spend a few moments each day preferably before your workout, using this exercise to psych yourself up.

STUMBLING BLOCKS

So why, if an activity can do all of these things, don't we all rush out and join in? Well, some of us do, but it's hard to get started and keep going until it becomes a habit. Also people may be embarrassed to be seen attempting something they may feel awkward at, or they may fear getting hurt or experiencing pain.

If you are disabled or have a limited range of motion, you may feel you cannot participate in activities that fully-abled people do. This is a misconception. There are ways to work around a disability for many sports and exercises. You may have to be a bit creative and, of course, you must consult your doctor before you begin, but provided you're in relatively good health, there should be no reason why you can't find some way to express your body in physical activity. I've seen people who are confined to a wheelchair or missing a limb ski, run marathons, swim, even play basketball. Don't let your limitations keep you from enjoying your body. You may have boundaries you must heed, but you can work within them to the fullest of your abilities.

The same concept applies to larger men and women. I'm fat, folks, but I dance, stretch, ride an exercise bike, wear outrageous clothes that look good on me, and have more and better sex than a lot of people I know. It's all part of my attitude. No, I can't go out and jog—the stress would be horrendous for my knees. I also am still recovering from an injury. But that doesn't prevent me from enjoying movement, or from believing that I can do so without looking foolish.

Still another stumbling block is the law of inertia. A body at rest will attempt to remain at rest unless acted upon from the outside. We may also believe that exercise must be boring or uncomfortable, or that we have to go over the top and work out every day. The truth is that a moderate amount of exercise several times a week is more than most people need to remain reasonably flexible and reap good benefits. If you want to increase your amount of exercise, do so gradually.

One of the most common reasons for failure to keep up with an exercise regimen is the crash-and-burn scenario. Flopsy decides to start an exercise program. She spends the first day or two on a nice even climb. Ten minutes, then fifteen minutes the second day. She feels good, so good in fact that she decides to boost it the third day to half an hour, and on the fourth and fifth days (if she makes it that long), she clocks in an hour. Come the weekend, her muscles catch up with her and she's in serious pain and can barely stretch out. By Monday, she still aches, is out of energy, and has decided that she's either not capable of going on, or she's leery of hurting herself any more than she already has. So she gives up and chalks it up to one more failure, thereby lowering her self-esteem and reinforcing the idea that she can't keep promises to herself.

During the '80s, women became exercise resistant. Since our society often links performance standards to exercise (competition/who is best/who is fastest, etc.), many women do not feel able to compete and continually compare themselves unfavorably to others. This can be true especially for those of us who were brought up in the era when women's sports were viewed as a joke; only men were *real* athletes outside of a few sports like gymnastics and tennis.

If you think you fall into this category, it is vital that you change your perception of exercise. Examine your feelings toward the subject, and if resistance comes up, perhaps you can find out what caused it. Since I was chubby when I was a young girl, I was laughed at a lot in school and always fell behind the other kids. I developed a deep anxiety due to gym class. Those were the days when thinness was simply considered a matter of will power.

I've been working on this slowly, trying not to compare myself to others as I move and exercise. It's a hard battle, one not easily overcome, but I know that eventually I'll be more at peace with the issue. I simply will not allow my self-esteem to fall as a result of past wrongs by ignorant people.

If you have to, consult a therapist on the issue. Exercise should be viewed as an enjoyable pursuit that is good for your body and health, rather than as a competition to be won or solely as a means to redesign your body. You are moving because your body is vibrant, because you need to stretch and move and play. Stagnation brings atrophy of both muscle and mind. Change ensures stability. Movement *is* life.

HOW TO FOCUS FOR SUCCESS

The key here is not to get caught in the burnout trap in the first place. How? Well, there are some ways you can trick yourself into success. First, you should schedule a physical with your doctor. She or he can tell you what you should be aware of when you begin an exercise program and can make you aware of health conditions that you should take into consideration. You should also consult your physician about what extra supplements you might need, though I strongly suggest you consider visiting a nutritionist, because quite often medical doctors are not schooled in anything beyond the basics in a proper diet.

For any exercise program to work, you must enjoy it. There's no mystery about this. If you do not enjoy what you're doing, you'll stop doing it. If you live in a cold climate but hate walking in cool weather, outdoor power walking is not likely to be of use to you. If you find routine annoying, don't take up a program that insists on the same format day after day. You'll need variation in your workout.

Some forms of exercise require a significant investment in gear and can easily become the basis for a shopping mania, so watch your pocketbook. While an initial outlay may be necessary—a piece of equipment or a good pair of shoes—you don't necessarily need to fork out a thousand bucks for a new workout wardrobe.

Do buy good shoes, however, if you choose any activity which requires foot support. It is vital that you find shoes that fit and are appropriate for the sport or activity you choose. Different muscles are needed for running than for basketball, and you will do yourself a favor if you invest in a pair of quality foot gear.

I find that if I exercise at nearly the same time every day, I have my best success. It becomes a habit. I try to break up my writing day to give my back a break from so much sitting down—writers are notorious for their back pain. Experts say it takes twenty-one days to create a habit. If you push yourself for three weeks, you have a much better chance of sticking to your workouts than you will if you are sporadic—another reason for making your workout mild to moderate for the first few weeks. If you do light stretching and a bit of dancing or biking each day, you won't wear yourself out and stumble into the burnout zone.

Try to approach your workout as if it were play. In a way, I dislike the term "workout," as it implies an unpleasant chore. If you can find the joy you had as a young child when the world was a toy box and there was nothing better than running around shrieking at the top of your lungs, you can recapture some of the joy you had in your body. Contrary to what our culture would like to believe, children are sensual beings and they know just how good it feels to run, to move, to touch themselves. We condition this joy out of them by imposing rules and regulations and telling them "Don't touch yourself there," and "No, you have to do it this way," and "You can't have a game without rules," to the point where we often remove all the fun from their play.

That happened to me with bowling. When I was little I really enjoyed it even though I couldn't roll the ball straight. But when someone tried to *teach* me how to bowl and began criticizing every move I made, I hated bowling and still do. Let your children enjoy their play. If they want to join a league or a group, they are going to have to learn the rules, but if they just want to have fun, encourage them to explore their own choice of movement. And if you were stifled in your physical expression as a child, take the time now to reacquaint yourself with the joy that your body can bring.

Some people like to chart their progress in a journal, while others find that they don't need to. You may want to experiment with a journal and see what works for you.

Combine exercise with decent food habits and you're going to find your energy level and confidence level shoot up. Isn't it worth the effort?

THE ZONE

Summer Solstice, 1991: I am dancing around the bonfire. This is the first Pagan festival I've been to, and so far I am in that blissful zone of feeling wild and free and in a group of people who understand me. The drums are pounding, the drummers are trancing out and their thunder echoes through the ground, through the air, through my body. People are dancing, drinking, making love, clapping their hands, howling at the moon. I love to dance, have danced for years, both in and out of ritual, but this is unlike any other experience. The drums speak to my blood, they call me out into the night, they move my feet. I have no self-consciousness about my size; I'm wearing a long, full black gauze skirt and a black halter top with red lace, and I feel beautiful.

I dance, I let my arms flow to the beat, I feel my hair whipping back and forth in the night. At one point my garnet necklace flies off my head to land in the grass beside me. After a quick break to grab it and drop it in my pack, I come back to the fire, swallow a long drink of cool water, and begin again. I follow the music, one beat, one thread in the thunderous, hypnotic force that drives the dancers on. I zero in on one of the musicians and begin to follow his beat alone. As I swing my body into the rhythm of his drumming, I look up and catch him staring at me. We lock eyes as I dance to the tattoo of his cadence. He intensifies the meter, drives it harder, and I react in turn, throwing myself fully into the music, still following his eyes.

We make love through the music, we fuck through the beat, he caresses me with his fingers as he caresses the skin of the drum. I soak in the driving thrust of his drumming and cycle it through me, then return it with my movements, reaching out to stroke his body through my gestures. The passion of the dance increases.

I am aware that there are others around doing the same thing. The drummers pick up on certain dancers who have that instinctive feel for the music. And then, as the echoes rebound around us, I feel myself lift and soar. I am both within my body, and outside of myself—I see from both vantage points. I feel my spirit lifting, touching the others who are in this intoxicating orgasm of movement, and then I feel the moon, the ground, the very air as it crackles with life, and I am part of that life, part of that ecstasy and joy.

Then, as the drums begin to soften, as the beat slows, I slowly reenter myself, soaked with sweat, limp, and thoroughly drained. I find a log, sit and drink water, close my eyes and then, as the drummers pick up a new beat, I am once again on my feet. I spend the night as part of the dance.

The next morning, men and women come up to me, thank me for dancing and for being so free to express myself. I do not realize until this moment how many people were watching—I was lost within the sound, not worrying about appearances, not worrying about my weight. I see once again how energy can shape the aura and influence people. The others give me hugs. I hug them back and smile. Now I understand that, yes, I am beautiful; because I allow myself to be who I am, I allow myself to experience joy in life. And I know that I want this feeling to continue. I want to be part of the cosmic dance of life, to transcend the chains I have built for myself through adhering to stereotypes.

The place where the body and spirit meet, where the body becomes an instrument for Divine connection, is a cosmic orgasm, if you will. You don't need to be part of a group like the one I was in. I've had that same "out-of-body/in-body" connection dancing alone or using a stationary bicycle.

As I mentioned earlier, when we exercise we produce endorphins that can trigger feelings of heightened awareness and extreme consciousness, but I think there's more involved in reaching this state. If you are approaching your exercise with the desire to connect to the Divine through bodywork, if you meditate before your workout, if you view your movement as a prayer, as a mantra, your attitude will alter the way your workout affects you.

When I dance, I view myself not as a dancer, but as part of the dance. By not separating myself from the movement, I become the movement and so remove the division between myself and the feeling. And when we remove that wall that keeps us insular in our experience, we also remove the barriers to enlightenment through the body. We are not seeking to forgo the body, we are not seeking *release* from it—we are seeking connection to the cosmic passion, the Divine marriage through the body. We simultaneously remain grounded and yet reach out to the universe, and blend both experiences to produce transcendence-in-body.

I focus on dance as being appropriate for this type of work, but I know other exercises and sports can lead to this connection. One reason I like the movement of dance to achieve this transcendent state is because of the music. Music affects not only our moods, but our bodies as well. The beat alters our heartbeat and changes the flow of our energy. The way we interact with the music can set up an hypnotic focus through which we can channel our energy. Of course, you can always use music with biking, stretching, etc. I find it a great motivator when I'm on an exercise bike; I just flow into the music and let my mind drift.

You probably won't reach this zone every time you exercise, but the more your body gets used to the movement, the more you can focus on the emotional and spiritual qualities of what you are doing, the less you will focus on trying to get the technique down.

CHAPTER SEVEN

Dancing, Yoga, and Exercise

Dance, dance, for the figure is easy,
The tune is catching and will not stop;
Dance till the stars come down from the rafters
Dance, dance, dance till you drop.

—W.H. Auden, "Death's Echo"

WARMING UP

While exercise should be play, as well as a discipline, we must learn how to avoid hurting ourselves. Before beginning any workout, you should warm up. Certain activities require stretches and light pre-workouts to get you ready for the stress you're about to put on your body. A good guideline is that ten minutes of light movement and gentle stretching will leave you limber enough to proceed. I recommend that you move and stretch according to what you are going to be doing. For instance, if you are dancing, you will want to warm up with light movements that will focus on loosening those muscles you'll be needing. I recommend a wonderful book, *Complete Stretching*, by Maxine Tobias and John Patrick Sullivan. It offers adjustments to certain exercises for those who are in need of modified movement. One thing I cannot abide is an exercise guide that assumes you are already in shape or lithe enough to maneuver yourself into any position. You can also buy some of the sports creams and apply them to your muscles before a workout. These help warm up the joints more quickly and will ease the amount of pain you will feel. Here are some other pointers:

- Don't bounce as you stretch; bouncing can tear the muscles if they are too cold.
- Make your movements smooth and fluid. When you reach for your toes, do so slowly and evenly, then grasp your ankles or toes. Do not bounce your head up and down toward your knees, just pull into the stretch slowly.
- Practice rhythmic breathing as you warm up to increase the flow of oxygen through your muscles. Do not hyperventilate.
- Wear loose clothing; remove all jewelry and your eyeglasses, if possible.
- Wait for a couple hours after a big meal before exercising.
- Try to get enough sleep. It will increase your performance.
- Do not force yourself past the pain barrier when you are warming up. You need to ease yourself slowly into a heavy-duty workout.
- Do not hold your breath when you are warming up. This will create tension and stress in your body. Breathe in a normal but rhythmic pattern.
- Gradually increase the pace of your warm-up until you are into the actual workout.
- Once you are warmed up, you can move on to your central exercise: yoga, dancing, weightlifting—anything that catches your imagination.

THE ART OF HATHA YOGA

The term "yoga" is derived from *yogah,* the Sanskrit word for *yoke* or *union.* Yoga is a 5,000-year-old Hindu discipline that involves using the body to train one's consciousness in order to reach spiritual insight.

Hatha yoga, the most common form of yoga in the Western world, means the union of the sun (*ha*) and the moon (*tha*), thereby creating a unified male/female, fire/water, yin/yang sense of self. Hatha yoga concerns itself primarily with the body through various *asanas* (exercises or postures). With a heavy emphasis on breath control, the goal is to bring the physical body into a perfect state of health and alignment.

An excellent method for relieving stress, Hatha yoga promotes strength, flexibility, and balance. With the long-term goal of bringing about inner peace and spiritual rejuvenation, this is one of the easiest exercises for people of all ages, shapes, and sizes to do. It can be tailored to your individual needs and can be used by those people with problems such as arthritis, fatigue, and high blood pressure.

One of the most important components of Hatha yoga is breath control, also known as *pranayama.* Rhythmic breath control can release the physical effects of stress and tension and promote better blood circulation. The increase in oxygen intake can only help your body, since most Americans (and perhaps those in other cultures) don't know how to breathe right. This increase in airflow heightens your ability to concentrate and focus.

The asanas of Hatha yoga have a revitalizing effect on your internal organs, as well as on your joints and flexibility. The movements create a conduit for energy to move through your body. Contrary to what most people think, Hatha yoga is not just a physical practice. It also awakens the Kundalini force.

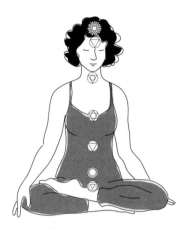

The seven major chakras

The Kundalini

The Kundalini force, the life force of our bodies and spirits, lies coiled at the base of our spine in our root or base chakra. There are seven major chakras up the back and front of the torso. They are power points, composing a system of energy. The base chakra is at the tailbone, and the crown chakra is on the top of the head. It is through these points that we run energy during sex magick or spiritually focused exercises.

Think of the Kundalini as a serpent embodying our life energy, passion, and creativity. It tends to remain dormant until awakened by meditation, energy work, or disciplines such as yoga. By gradually arousing the serpent within, we expand our consciousness and achieve a communion with the Divine.

There is a discipline known as Kundalini yoga, but I would advise that you first become proficient in Hatha yoga. If you awaken the Kundalini too fast, you may find yourself in trouble, for the intensity of the forces unleashed can be overwhelming. I've read reports of people who have been ridden as if by a Voudoun Loa during the awakening of their Kundalini. You may also find that as you progress, your libido will kick into overdrive. During their thirties and forties, many women commonly find their sex drive dramatically increases. When you combine that with the rising Kundalini, you may feel at times that you're becoming a nymphomaniac. There are days when I could have sex all day long and still be ready for more. You cannot awaken the Kundalini in one area of your life—such as exercise or meditation—and not have it affect the rest of your life. So be aware that you are dealing with the primal life force here, the fire of Shiva and Shakti, and it can and will affect you. Earthly passion is one thing; Divine passion another.

Once you have begun to awaken the Kundalini, you must not try to shove it back down the spine or repress it. You must work through the energies that it rouses and learn to integrate them into your life. There's no turning back after you open the psychic senses within. Repression leads to all manner of physical, emotional, and psychic illnesses and mishaps, but if you go at an even pace and honestly gauge your abilities, you should be fine.

SOME BASIC ASANAS AND MEDITATION PRACTICES

Here are a few basic asanas. These are only the bare bones; I encourage you to check out the bibliography at the back of this book, where I've included several good books as well as some videos that will help guide you. I've included one video title that is geared toward larger people and proves once again that you don't have to be thin to be healthy and fit.

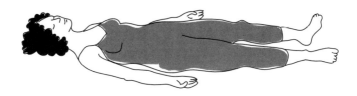

The Salvasana (Deep Relaxation Posture)

Almost everyone recognizes the Lotus posture, but it is only one of many, and not all body types will be comfortable in the full Lotus. Therefore, we will start with a posture that just about anyone can do. For this asana, you must put aside thoughts of conventional exercise. Lie on the floor on your back and close your eyes. Take three deep breaths and slowly exhale as you allow your body to go limp.

Focus on your feet and legs. Feel for any tension. If you find any, tense that area, then relax and let it go limp. Move up into your groin, your torso, and your arms, repeating the tensing and relaxing in each area. Go slowly, breathing deeply and slowly. Do not hyperventilate. When you reach your head and have relaxed your neck, remain in this peaceful state for one to two minutes, listening to your breath.

Energy work: When you have reached the state of complete relaxation, feel for your aura which surrounds your body. Can you sense how far the energy extends from your skin? Do you see or sense a color? Does it feel different when you are relaxed or when you are in a rush or stressed out?

Now slowly sit up and go on to your other asanas.

Pranayama (Complete Breath)

There is a difference between shallow breathing and deep breathing. In this exercise, you will breathe with your diaphragm, which allows you to breathe deeply. Any singer or belly dancer will tell you that singing and dancing effectively depends on learning to breathe from the diaphragm and control its movements.

Sit in a cross-legged position or stand, slightly bent at the hips, with your hands resting on your thighs or a chair. For this posture, you will be breathing through your nose, filling your lungs with air. Take a slow deep breath through your nose and hold it to a count of five. Feel your stomach expand. It helps to keep one hand on your abdomen during this learning phase, so you can feel your breath contract and expand. Hold your breath for a count of five, then slowly exhale through your mouth, again to the count of five. You should now feel your stomach contract. When you've expelled the air from your lungs, hold for a count of five. Repeat for a total of five full breaths.

Energy work: When you have become comfortable with this asana, start focusing on the energy that you raise by breathing this way. See the energy as a wave that flows in and then ebbs out. Draw in energy from the air surrounding you. Run it through your body, down your windpipe, and into your lungs, then push the wave up and out through your mouth. The *prana,* or breath energy, cleanses and recharges as it slides down into your lungs and deep into your body. When it exits through your mouth, it takes with it stagnation and feelings of lethargy and fatigue.

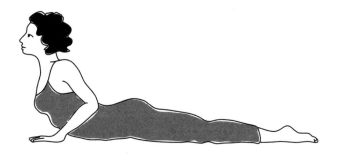

Bhujangasana: The Cobra

The Cobra is a very beneficial stretch for the back. Lie on your stomach with your elbows bent to your sides, hands flat on the floor under your chest. Rest your head on the mat or rug and let your body relax. Breathe rhythmically at an even pace.

Slowly begin to push your torso up with your hips and groin still touching the floor. With a smooth movement, use your hands to push your upper torso into an arch slowly, so that your head is up, your eyes are forward, and your spine is curved. If you cannot manage this extreme stretch at first, go as far as you comfortably can. Hold this position for a count of ten, then slowly lower yourself to the floor. Repeat five times.

Energy work: As you rise up, feel yourself become the Cobra. Picture the Kundalini force traveling up your spine as you stretch, feel it arching as it creeps up your back, just as the King Cobra arches, and visualize it fountaining out of your crown chakra, showering you with a radiant light.

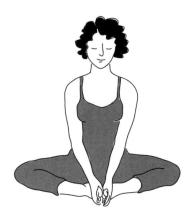

Bhadrasana: The Butterfly

The Butterfly asana will not only give your legs a good stretch, it will prepare you for the Lotus. Sit on the floor; you may wish to sit on a thin cushion to facilitate this at first. Gently stretch your legs out in front of you, spreading them slightly. First bend one knee, then the other, and touch the bottom of your soles together.

Slide your soles as close to your groin as you comfortably can, and grasp your feet with your hands. Gently lower your knees as far to the floor as you can without straining. Hold this position for a slow count of thirty, then stretch your legs out in front of you. Repeat five times.

Energy work: As you sit in the Butterfly position, visualize a circle of energy running from your base chakra up your spine. Feel it travel down your right side into your right leg, and from there into the sole of your right foot. Allow the energy to transfer into the sole of your left foot. Bring the energy up through the left leg and back up into your crown chakra. Then circle the energy in the opposite direction—from your crown chakra down the left side, through the left foot into the

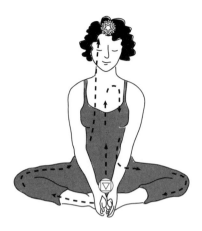

right, and then back up into the crown chakra. Do not take the energy back down the spine into the base chakra.

The examples should give you some idea of what the yoga asanas can do for you. You can develop the energy work as you practice them. It is important to remember that once the Kundalini is aroused, you should not try to take it back down your spine—you could throw yourself out of balance and impede your progress. Repression is not an option here.

DANCING

In the last chapter, I talked about my experiences dancing at Pagan festivals, and how I made love with the drummer through the music, through the movement. I find that dancing lends itself to the passion of raising the Kundalini, of freeing the soul to journey into the sphere of the Divine. There's something about the blend of hypnotic music, of body-in-motion, of feeling every note flow into the core of your heart that opens up the senses and allows you to soar.

There are several forms of dance you can choose, or you can just express yourself in movement. *Bellydancing*, or Middle Eastern dancing, is a beautiful art form which has an extremely wide following within both the Pagan community and the general community. Most of the music used is hypnotic and can lull you deep within yourself, and the dance itself can help you form a spiritual connection to your body. There are different forms of bellydance, and although some of them have been turned into a "shake your boobs for the men" show, bellydancing remains one of the most pleasant ways to celebrate and express your sexuality. I've seen extremely talented male bellydancers, so it's not just for women.

Middle Eastern dance is often used to entertain and amuse friends and relatives, and to celebrate joyful events. We can also speculate that it or something similar (ancient Egypt and Africa both had a similar form of dance) may have been used to celebrate holy days and invoke the gods.

Some of the basic maneuvers in bellydancing are extraordinarily good for digestion, and for muscle tone in the waist, hips, and thighs. The muscle control required of the diaphragm is exquisite and not all that difficult to master with proper concentration. One of the wonderful things about this dance is that it is meant for curvaceous female bodies. In other words, large women can be extremely good bellydancers. Size isn't a factor; what's important is the ability to be comfortable in your body, to learn graceful, sinuous movements, and to focus on the music.

I recommend the video, *Bellydance! Magical Motion with Atéa*, if you are interested in learning the basics. Though all the dancers in the video are rather thin, I had no trouble learning the moves from them, and Atéa moves at a comfortable pace. Do what you can, and the next time, try to do a bit more. The costuming in the video is lovely.

Hula

You might also wish to look into the practice of hula, as taught by a true *kumu hula* (hula teacher). When performed for the right reasons, hula is a gift to the gods, an offering of love and joy, a retelling of ancient tales. There are strict forms of hula, especially *hula kahiko* or the ancient hula, which is based on the drum and chant rather than on the ukulele and song.

When most people think of hula, they think of ukuleles, grass skirts, and women whose hips move faster than a propeller blade. They think of luxurious hotels and luaus and movies like *South Pacific*. But the art of hula is far older than Hawaii's entrance into Western culture and far more sacred.

An integrated combination of movement, *mele* (poetry), and rhythm, hula originated as both a tribute to the gods and a way to preserve history. Seldom used as entertainment, the dances were passed down through the generations in strict form, for this was the Hawaiians' way of recording their past and paying tribute and respect to the gods. If you altered the dance or performed it without the utmost devotion or concentration, you would change history and show the gods your lack of concern.

Hula was also used to commemorate specific events, such as the birth of a royal child or the onset of war, and there are indications that it was used in magic, in rites for fertility or abundance.

Hula is taught within a *halau* (school) by a *kumu* (teacher). There are both *'olapa* (the dancers) and *ho'opa'a* (the chanters and percussionists). While the hula may be performed without instruments, historically the dance was never performed without chanting or singing.

When Christian missionaries arrived in Hawaii in the 1820s, they were scandalized by the Pagan rites and rituals. Hula was seen as a sexual rather than a ceremonial practice and was branded as sinful. The missionaries couldn't accept the scant clothing or uninhibited nature of the Hawaiians and quickly set out to abolish the hula. When Queen Ka'ahumanu, widow of Kamehameha I, was baptized a Christian, she outlawed public performance of the hula. This edict broke up the stronghold of the halau and effectively started the destruction of one of the oldest practices on the islands.

When David Kalakaua took the throne in 1874, he instigated a resurgence of interest in Hawaiian culture. Nicknamed the "Merrie Monarch," he rescinded the edict forbidding the hula and encouraged the renewed pursuit of the dance. He built the 'Iolani Palace and instituted an orchestra that played every day for public enjoyment. Though there were fifty years between the hula of the past and the hula of Kalakaua's time, the dance was alive once more.

However, hula had now become more of an entertainment. Ritual and ceremonial roots were ignored and Westerners began using it as a tourist gimmick. "See the beautiful Hawaiian girls wiggle their hips," and so on. As the century turned and Hawaii's monarchy was overthrown by the United States, the dance was co-opted and turned into burlesque. Through the machinations of Hollywood, the beautiful Hawaiian hula girl became the basis for such movies as *South Pacific,* Elvis's *Blue Hawaii,* and numerous other films. Luxury hotels promoted all forms of Polynesian dance as hula and lumped them together in Westernized versions of luaus, further taking the hula down to the level of pure entertainment.

Still, underneath all the cellophane skirts and plastic leis, something of the old form remained. Then in the 1970s, a renewed interest in the culture and religion of Hawaii brought the ancient kahiko form back into the spotlight. As foundations and organizations arose to document, preserve, and perpetuate Hawaiian history, hula halaus once again blossomed and the ancient traditions, modified for this century, were reinstated.

Today the debate still rages, however, on whether kahiko hula should stand as it once stood without alteration or change, or whether some of the new dances, created in the kahiko style, are acceptable additions to the ever-growing body of legend and mele behind the form.

In Hawaii, there are specific goddesses to whom the hula is sacred. Laka, the foremost goddess and creatrix of the dance, demanded strict *kapu* (or taboos) regarding certain actions during hula training. Breaking these kapu resulted in swift and direct punishment, and students took the chance of offending the Goddess if they succumbed to temptation. Laka's kapu included sex, unhygienic practices, disrespect to the teacher, and other infractions. Rituals to purify the student after breaking kapu had to be performed before the dancer would be back in the good graces of the kumu, the halau, and the Goddess.

While Laka is considered the primary patroness of the hula throughout many of the legends, Hi'iaka embodies the spirit of the dance. There is a tremendous body of work recounting the sagas of Hi'iaka and her older sister, Pele. Over three hundred songs and chants record the epic struggle between Pele and Hi'iaka over the ho'opa'a Lohi'au.

The primary story of Pele and Hi'iaka centers around a young chanter named Lohi'au, with whom Pele has fallen in love. Lohi'au is a mortal who resides on the island of Kaua'i, and Pele misses him dearly. She asks Hi'iaka to fetch him for her and Hi'iaka agrees, asking in return that Pele protect her 'ohi'a lehua groves while she's gone. Pele gives Hi'iaka forty days to complete the journey.

The meles tell of Hi'iaka's exploits as she sets about her task, and the people she meets along the way. Using cunning and magic, Hi'iaka manages to field her way through the various evil spirits that dwell throughout the island chain, and reaches Lohi'au's side. Unfortunately, a rift occurs between the two sisters when it takes Hi'iaka more than forty days to complete her task and, though she is loyal to her sister and refrains from sleeping with the attractive Lohi'au, Pele suspects her and flies into a jealous rage. She sends her fires and lava down to destroy Hi'iaka's sacred groves.

As Hi'iaka and Lohi'au return to the Big Island, Hi'iaka sees her groves charred and burned, and in revenge retaliates by embracing Lohi'au in front of Pele. Pele attacks, covering them with lava. While her sister cannot be harmed because she is a goddess, Lohi'au is burnt to a crisp. One of Pele's brothers who witnessed this battle catches hold of the spirit of Lohi'au and returns him to his body. Lohi'au and Hi'iaka are reunited and return to Kauai.

Another story tells of Pele's volatile love affair with Kamapua'a, the Hawaiian Pig God who follows her everywhere, wooing her even as she insults him, calling him a pig. Their arguments build until Kamapua'a's rage erupts in torrential rainstorms while Pele retaliates by opening the earth and pouring rivers of lava over his forests. Eventually, Kamapua'a's storms begin to quench Pele's sacred fires. Fearing that she will lose the battle, Pele's brothers order her to sleep with the Pig God. She acquiesces and they become on-again off-again lovers, always fighting, always arguing, and yet passionately embracing one another as their lust fills the islands with energy and vibrancy.

The hulas that retell these stories are beautiful to watch—but when performed with devotion and concentration, the energy and mana that the dancers raise is noticeable even through a television set.

Every year, there are numerous hula competitions that people can attend. The Merrie Monarch competition, named after King Kalakaua, is probably the most prestigious in the world. Performers are judged not only on their performance, but on their costume, expression, and the mana they bring to the dance. If you ever have the chance to attend, you will not regret it.

Hula as a spiritual dance requires the will to submit to the teacher, to learn the patterns and movements without imposing your own style. It is truly a dance for those who are willing to prostrate themselves before the gods, to follow tradition, and be honorable to the codes that the various halau require.

I have spent hours watching the dances of hula kahiko, and each time I am as mesmerized as I was on my first viewing. The spiritual energy is palpable within the form.

Trance Dancing

I tend to get most of my exercise through trance dancing. I have studied a little bellydancing, a little hula; I've practiced yoga in strict form. I've lifted weights and worked with a stationary bike. And always, always, I come back to trance dancing. A type of free-form dancing, what I call trance dancing includes moves from all the different forms I've seen or studied, including yoga.

I work with music from Dead Can Dance, Gabrielle Roth and the Mirrors, Tangerine Dream, and bellydancing music from CDs such as *Eternal Egypt.* My first ten minutes or so are spent in free-form, slow-motion movement to the music in order to stretch my muscles and get them warmed up. I let myself slide into the music, feel it enter my blood, feel the pulse in my heart. Starting with head and shoulder rolls, I move in time to the rhythms, let my body sink into the beat. After my neck and shoulders are loosened up, I move on to my arms, spine, hips, legs, knees, and feet. I make this one continuous series of movements, never stopping, flowing from one warm-up to another, all with a slow and rhythmic breath and at an even pace. I usually pick a warm-up song like "Indus" (Dead Can Dance: *Spiritchaser*) that is about ten minutes long to guide me.

When this part of the dance is over, I move on to floor work, lowering myself, and again in rhythm, I stretch my legs, my back, etc., all with a continual flow. By this time, I'm captivated by the beat of the music and fully involved in feeling it run through my body. This phase takes about another ten to fifteen minutes.

In the third phase, I rise and begin a faster movement—free-form—combining bellydancing, hula movements, and the sense of my body responding to the music. I let the melody guide my arms; I let my feet flow into the harmony and become the pulse, the drum, the flute that wavers, the chant. It's all a prayer, all a vision of love and reverence, of reaching for that Divine spark with the body, lifting myself to the status of a temple in which I pray and reach out to the macrocosm.

I drift in this phase, transform it into a moving meditation, a vision of energy swirling within me as I swirl within the fire of the universe. Keep moving, keep the body in motion, for the motion brings creation. Leave all daily care and worry; I am more than mere dancer, I am part of the whole, part of the dance of the universe, and I may meet Shakti or Shiva gliding through the heavens as they dance the world into creation.

Breathe deep, inhale, breathe in the force of creation. As I exhale, the breath removes all stagnation from my body. I become the dance.

There is no right or wrong here. There is no need for a class, a guru, or a mentor. All we need is the music, the will, and the ability to put our egos aside, to step outside ourselves so that we can connect with the Divine. Once we let go, once we walk away from the "I" and give ourselves up to the dance, we are so much more than we ever thought we could be. We are stars twinkling in the night sky, we are patterns of the kaleidoscope, we are grains in the sand painting of the monk. And here we enter the zone.

COOLING DOWN

After you reach the peak of your exercise (which will sometimes be more intense than others), you will need to cool down. You can return to the light stretching you did during the warm-up, or you can walk slowly for about five minutes until your breath returns to normal. If you do not cool down, you risk injuring your body by abruptly stopping your movements. I also suggest ending each session with a brief meditation.

Returning-to-Body Meditation

After you have cooled down, stand barefoot in a comfortable stance and close your eyes. Take three slow, deep breaths and let any remaining tension exit your body. Focus your attention on your feet. Feel the floor beneath them. You have roots that delve deep into the floor, through wood and concrete, through dirt and stone, to the center of the world. Your roots burrow down; they dig into the bowels of the world, into the core. Let them gather energy and sustenance from the body of the Earth Mother upon whose back we walk. Feel your connection to her, take a deep breath, and give a prayer of thanks for your life, for your blessings.

Now take three slow, deep breaths. Focus your attention on your hands and raise them over your head. Feel the air surrounding them. You radiate a light that shines upward, that spirals toward the sky, toward the heavens to reach the sky and the stars beyond. Feel the spirals from your hands gather energy from the celestial realms within which our minds roam. Feel your connection to those Devi who wander the skies. Take a deep breath, and give a prayer of thanks for your life, for your blessings.

Now bring your attention to your base chakra where your Kundalini resides. See the chakra as a lotus, opening and brilliant, radiating passion and creativity, life and love, fire and vision. Feel your connection to your own self, take a deep breath, and give a prayer of thanks for your life, for your blessings.

You may open your eyes when you are ready.

MASSAGE

One of the best ways to help your body recover from exercise and stress is through massage. I have always loved having my back, arms, and feet rubbed, but until I started going to a massage therapist, I didn't fully realize how many benefits a good, professional massage could bring.

As with any health care professional, you should feel comfortable with your masseuse. You should clarify what you want from the massage. Be realistic about how much can be done in one session. I knew my muscles were strained, but I didn't realize just how tight and painful they had become. Kellie Robertson, my massage therapist, found adhesions (two or more muscle tissues which are normally separate, but which had fused together) everywhere. She discovered that what I had thought of as simply good solid muscle was tight, unmovable muscle. Initially I thought, "I'm in need of some work on my body"; I left knowing that I was in need of a full-scale, ongoing series of treatments.

Kellie and I have talked about what massage can and can't do. Because it was easy to sense the care and the value she puts into her work, I decided an interview with her would be an interesting addition to this book.

INTERVIEW WITH KELLIE ROBERTSON, MASSEUSE

Yasmine: Tell me a bit about yourself.

Kellie: I'm twenty-eight years old, single, and have a dog and a cat. I graduated from college in 1997 with a Bachelor's of Fine Arts, emphasizing ceramics. I love to work with my hands. I moved to

Seattle from Denver because my brother, sister-in-law, and their new baby lived here. I didn't like Denver and I really like being close to my family.

Yasmine: How long have you been a massage therapist (MT) and how did you become one?

Kellie: When I moved to Seattle, I was working as a baker at a fine restaurant and was pursuing ceramics during my spare time. But it wasn't fulfilling enough. I realized I couldn't work at just any job to sustain my art and also knew the restaurant field wasn't for me. When my dad told me about my cousin who was thinking of becoming an MT, I thought, "I could do that."

When I make pottery, I want the person viewing the finished piece to feel good about it, to take pleasure in the beauty of the work. Similarly, there are a lot of stressed-out people in the world and I like helping them feel good about themselves. I like helping them get in touch with their bodies.

Yasmine: When did you first realize you had an interest in massage therapy? Have you always considered yourself a form of healer?

Kellie: I realized that I was interested in MT when I couldn't imagine myself working behind a desk, as a waitress or teacher. Those jobs just don't give me enough spiritually. I wanted to help people feel good, but couldn't think how I could do that. This way, I can achieve my goal while being my own boss.

Have I always considered myself a form of healer? I wouldn't say that. I have always been easy to talk to. I make people comfortable. I can't say I'm a spiritual healer except that I listen to people and let them talk about whatever may be on their minds. Talking lets feeling come out, rather than repressing it and letting it work against us on the inside. I would say that in this way I help people heal themselves.

Yasmine: A lot of people don't realize massage is so complicated. Tell me a little about your schooling. Why did you choose to learn the forms of massage you did?

Kellie: The massage school I chose had a twelve-month program split into four terms. The classes included anatomy, physiology, kinesiology (the study of muscles and why they work), massage theory, and practice. We had specific classes for pregnancy, sports, chronic pain, and hydrotherapy. Each term, we also had classes in business, legal stuff, taxes, and invoices. During our third term we were required to work in the student clinic, and during our fourth term we had the choice between continuing to work in the student clinic or going on to an outside internship. We had special projects we had to finish, and we also learned CPR and took an HIV/AIDS course. Our finals covered everything we had learned over the twelve-month period in order to prepare us for the state board exams.

The foundation for all the techniques we learned is Swedish massage and relaxation massage. The school I attended focuses on treatment work. When I graduated, I decided to emphasize relaxation massage.

One of the things I like about being a licensed masseuse is that licensed MTs have to take classes in order to retain their licenses. This requirement can only enhance the experience for both my client and myself.

Yasmine: Massage is a very intimate form of contact. How do you cope with being so involved with a stranger's body?

Kellie: Massage can be a very intimate form of contact, yes, but intention is everything. As an MT, my intention is to help clients relax, feel comfortable with me touching them (appropriately always), help them get in touch with their own bodies, and realize the changes they go through during the massage.

Yasmine: I believe that massage can have a spiritual form—working through the aura. How do you view this side of it? Do you find that your energy changes depending on whom you are working with?

Kellie: I pick up on energy very easily—other people's and the room in general. With some clients I can work through their energy faster than I can with others. Let me explain. I put my hands over their feet first, or I put my hands over their heads. This could be the place they've been all day. I wait until their energy lets me touch them. It's like a wall; when the wall is down, we can begin the massage. My own energy changes depending on who I'm working with. So far, I've managed to stay very positive.

Yasmine: Talk a little bit about ideal clients. What attitude should they bring to the table to help you help them?

Kellie: Ideal clients are people who are open to massage. They are there to relax, yet they go into their body and the experience of the massage. They will notice and observe the changes their body goes through as it relaxes.

Yasmine: Now, on the flip side, what kind of client makes you cringe?

Kellie: The client who makes me cringe has the idea that the massage is sexual and acts a little too friendly. When this happens, I just put on my professional face and let the client know that the massage is in no way going to be or should be sexual. We can then continue on this basis or the client can find another MT.

Yasmine: Have you refused to massage some people? What brought you to that decision?

Kellie: I have refused one person so far. He had a heart attack three days prior to the massage. One of the effects of massage therapy is that it increases your heart rate, then lowers it. I can't put that added stress on someone who is obviously in some danger or risk from a massage. He would have to have a written approval from his doctor beforehand.

Yasmine: There are many types of bodies. Have you found you had to get over any blocks about body size, shape, color? If so, how did you cope with this?

Kellie: When I first became interested in massage, my biggest fear was having to deal with a large, hairy man on my table who had an erection [*laughs*]. Luckily, my school takes such fears very seriously and taught us how to deal with such situations. Now I know a body is just a body, whatever the size, shape, or color. I like working with people. It's fascinating to feel and see the differences in body types.

Yasmine: What makes you happiest during a massage? I know you've talked to me about how much you enjoy seeing clients progress in their bodywork—can you elaborate on that?

Kellie: I like to make people feel mushy—totally relaxed. I also really enjoy the sensation when a muscle relaxes. It will be tight and congested one second, then it releases, and the tension dissipates. I enjoy my work even more when my clients and I work together (by having them breathe slowly and deeply) because they will then be able to feel that release too and understand a bit more about how their bodies work.

Yasmine: What do you advise people to look for in a masseuse? What kind of questions do you wish people would ask you?

Kellie: When looking for an MT, you should see how well the two of you click. How does the energy feel? There is nothing worse than getting a massage from someone you can't stand. Listen to what the masseuse says about the type of massage he or she practices. When people ask me, I tell them the basics. If they seem more interested, I go into more detail about the depth of the massage, pain, and the communication that there must be between us as client and therapist.

If they choose to get a massage from me and like it—that's wonderful. If they don't enjoy it—well, not everyone will like my techniques. I tell people to take what they like from my massage and then ask the next MT they interview whether any other practices are included in the massage.

One thing I must stress: if the MT does something that hurts or doesn't feel good, say something! The MT should stop and adjust what he or she is doing. Do ask about draping—is there any, how is it done, and what parts of the body stay covered?

Yasmine: Sometimes people have high expectations about body-work—what it can do and the speed with which it can make changes in their bodies. Talk a little about what you can and cannot expect from massage therapy.

Kellie: You need to be aware of the shape your body is in when you first come to see an MT. It's going to take some time to undo the damage. If the client is ready to be patient, if the client keeps up with the sessions, does the stretches, and drinks lots of water, he or she will see improvement. It takes time to undo the harm that stress, trauma, injury, etc. put on the body. And remember, each individual will react differently to massage.

Yasmine: I know that you've helped me a lot already and I'm looking forward to seeing what shape my body is in six months from now.

CARVING TIME OUT FOR YOUR EXERCISE

When you begin to exercise, you will probably find it necessary to slow yourself down consciously. Most of us today tend to be constantly on the move. We feel that we aren't getting enough done; we load up our schedules until we are at the point of exhaustion. Got to move faster—need more time, more space, more money. Now to some extent, we can't help this; we live in a world that moves rapidly. However, we can do something to regain some equilibrium.

Do you really need to have a spotless house? You do? Then if you have kids, enlist their help; chores are good for them. I'm a major proponent of technology: dishwashers, washers, dryers, whatever you can find to make your life a bit less stressful. Can you accumulate errands until you can spend one afternoon a week on them, rather than running out every day and wasting time?

Live too far from your work? Can you move closer? Commuting eats up so many hours for many people. When my husband got his new job this year, he was commuting 80 miles a day each way. Even though we liked the city we lived in, the situation was ridiculous. Once we'd made the move to our new home closer to his work, it was much easier.

I used to shop once a month and stock up on everything. However, I've realized that by doing so, I spent more time trying to plan our meals and putting away groceries than if I shopped once or twice a week for food. Arranging a month's food into thirty days worth of meals boggled my mind, and the way I must eat now, it makes no sense to buy in bulk, except for the stuff I can buy on sale and toss in the freezer.

Take a look at your life and see if there are ways you can streamline it without feeling you are shortchanging yourself. By rearranging your schedule, you might find you are able to take some pressure off.

When you carve out time for yourself to practice yoga or just to rest, you may find your guilt kicking in. You must learn to let go of this mechanism. If you don't put yourself first, if you don't take care of yourself, how can you possibly take care of anyone else? Keep yourself healthy, and you will have the strength to cope with everyday problems.

THE WALL

When I practiced yoga regularly, I noticed that when I was starting to make progress, I would rebel and quit. A month later I would berate myself, be back at it, and once again build up and quit.

I think that this stems from the fact that the muscles and the body as a whole have memory. When we first start an exercise program, we shock our systems. Our bodies think, "What the hell is this? You have got to be kidding!" And then our bodies humor us in the hope that we'll soon tire of this, come to our senses, and knock it off. As we make headway, as we go through day after day stretching or dancing or whatever, as the weeks pile up, our bodies begin to suspect that this isn't just a passing fancy. They are used to a particular state of being and have settled into atrophy. When our bodies realize we're serious, they begin applying the pressure and we find ourselves hitting the wall. "I can't do my workout today, simply can't because (fill in the blank)." Sound familiar? It's all too familiar to me because I've said it all too many times. No matter how much I love the work or how good it makes me feel, I hit the wall and come out with a nosebleed.

Some days you will have a cold or cramps or the flu and then, of course, you should use your common sense and stay in bed or rest rather than taxing your system any further. But how many of those days are you truly sick? How many times is your body or mind protesting because (gasp) this time you might actually succeed in your goal? The body knows that success brings with it the feeling that you must continue, that you must now move beyond the bare beginnings into new and unfamiliar territory.

This happens with everything. I hit the wall in my writing for a long time, until I decided I was willing to accept the success and responsibility that went with it. I've seen other people do the same in love relationships, careers, and bodywork. The wall is an invisible barrier through which we do not believe we can pass, or we're afraid to pass, afraid to venture into unknown territory.

How can you move beyond the wall? How can you tame the inner demons that whisper in your ears? We will examine various ways to cope with our fears of success, our fears of failure, and our body's resistance.

First, you have to be ready to make a change in your life. If you aren't ready, no amount of encouragement, help, focus, or magick in the world will aid you. I find over and over that people come to me for help but have a million reasons why every single thing I or anyone else suggests won't work. I no longer have patience for these people—they aren't ready to change and they don't really want to do the work. They want the results handed to them on a silver salver and refuse to make any effort that might be required of them. I refuse to waste my energy on these people.

Once you are ready to make a change, you must accept that change will likely be gradual, that you will have to work for what you get, and that the results may not be exactly what you envision. Often when you do decide to get a move on, you become impatient. "Why won't this happen faster? Why do I have to go through so much to get what I want?" Remember that it probably took months, even years, to reach the state you are presently in. You cannot possibly expect instantaneous change or even change within a week or a month. You might see fast progress, and in the case of exercise you will definitely notice an effect after a week or two. But long-term changes in health, body shape, and spirit will take a while.

When you come to grips with the fact that change is a gradual affair and that you will see results but no miracles for months to come, how do you avoid hitting the wall that causes so many good intentions to come to a halt? My advice is to take it one day at a time, one hour at a time.

I'm currently undergoing a radical change in diet. My aunt was recently diagnosed with severe hereditary Type 2 diabetes. I have low blood sugar, which increases my risk of developing the same disease. I have had to cut out sugar, reduce certain carbohydrates, and eat protein at every meal. For someone who is a sugar freak, and who already had to stop eating wheat, this is not easy. But I do not want diabetes, and I want to feel healthy. So I take the sugar cravings an hour at a time. Eventually they'll fade away. Until then, I grit my teeth and remember why I'm doing this.

Find a support system, a few good friends whom you can turn to if you are discovering a resistance within yourself. Exercise with someone who understands what you are aiming for and why. Make sure that your friends are not going to compete with you—that only leads to frustration. Instead, choose friends who will support you fully, make you feel competent about what you are doing, and tell you straight what you need to hear.

Record your progress. It's hard to overlook three weeks worth of check marks on a chart that indicate your progress.

Start slowly. Once again, it's better to begin small and grow, than it is to institute a grand change and burn out. Be content with baby steps to start with. You will advance toward your goal much faster that way.

COPING WITH INJURY

I stepped out of my car on July 11, 1994, into a dimly lit parking lot. It was one o'clock in the morning, and we were packing for a trip to Hawaii. My mother-in-law had sent us tickets. What a chance! We had so little money, we would never have been able to afford the trip on our own. As I shut the car door and turned, I stepped into a hole hidden in the darkness and fell.

At the emergency room, they told me it was a bad sprain. They wrapped it up and sent me home on crutches. The walk from the car to the apartment, which normally took less than five minutes, extended into an agonizing twenty. I had not only sprained my ankle, I had ripped tendons and ligaments all around my foot. By the time I managed my way into the apartment, I thought I was going to scream, and the pain pills they gave me didn't help; they only made me woozy.

The next day I received a phone call from the hospital—they had re-examined the x-ray and found a chip in my ankle bone. I should go to an orthopedist and have it set in a cast. Except there was one minor problem: we didn't have insurance and we didn't have the money for a cast. Moreover, the orthopedists I called required cash up front. We had no one to turn to, and I figured if it was a hairline fracture, it should heal quickly. So I wrapped my ankle up tight and we went to Hawaii as planned. I learned to grit my teeth with the pain. I also learned just how negligent this society is in its provisions for the disabled.

Instead of being on crutches for eight weeks, as I thought I would be, I was on crutches for over a year. After that, I spent three years in agony whenever I walked. My lower back burned like fire and my knees hurt so badly that I could barely carry a plate from my office into the kitchen. Samwise took over most of the chores to help me out, and we kept thinking that if I just could get enough stretching, it would be okay.

This was a dark time. I lived in shadows, but even as my anger grew, so did my ability to dive within, and there I discovered the ability and will to write my nonfiction magickal work. I also found out that some of my friends weren't willing to stick around when I was no longer able to run with the pack.

Just as I despaired of ever being able to function normally again, I remembered going to a chiropractor when I was a little girl and seeing how he helped my mother after a fall. I asked around, found two friends who went to the same man, and within ten minutes of my first visit, I was standing straight again for the first time in four years. But my progress has been slow—four years with a pinched nerve due to a hip that is out of joint doesn't heal overnight.

Then I discovered recently that I had edema around my joints and was put on diuretics. Within a few days, the swelling was down and a lot of the extra pain was gone. I've also began to get professional massages, another step in my recovery. And with the dancing that I do, I know that eventually I will be strong again. But it's hard to wait, and coping with pain has not been easy.

Chances are if you get injured you probably won't be laid up as I was. However, take a few tips from one who's been there: have your injury tended to. Beg or borrow the money if you have to. It isn't worth the pain of years of side effects from not getting proper medical attention. Meanwhile, bitch at your congressperson about the need for socialized/national health care. Too many people end up with problems because they simply cannot afford the medical care that requires cash up front.

Ease back into your workouts. Be cautious about strenuous activity soon after an injury. Consult your doctor about how soon you can resume your full schedule. Stretching, however, is always good for body parts that aren't injured.

Remember the keys to healing: RICE: *R*est, *I*ce, *C*ompression, and *E*levation. This is the formula used by doctors and physical therapists to enhance the healing of ankle sprains. Never ice an ankle for more than twenty minutes at a time unless directed to do so by your doctor, and always keep the ice wrapped in a towel. I've found that, for minor strains and aches, a bag of frozen peas works best—it conforms to the shape of the body part more easily than a stiff ice pack and isn't too heavy on the bruise. When you wrap an injured limb, never wrap it so tightly that the circulation is constricted.

The biggest obstacle when coping with injury can be emotional stress. When we're laid up and don't have full mobility, we tend to find our self-esteem plunging. It can be a struggle to keep our spirits up and our self-confidence intact when we need help for even simple tasks. Unfortunately, we may not feel okay about asking for help. We connect the concept of being a strong, independent person with being in top physical shape. Unless we have full mobility and are thin, young, and vibrant, we feel vulnerable and less than desirable. Unless we can run a lap every morning, spend half an hour on the treadmill in the afternoon, and go hiking up Rock Canyon at night, we feel we won't be able to live life to the fullest.

This is a shame. Sue Alcorn, whom I interviewed in chapter 3, is one of my closest online friends. She is disabled due to a muscular degeneration disease. She recently moved to a housing complex for the disabled and is fully capable of running her own life and taking care of her own needs. As someone who once had full mobility, she's been through the wringer with operation after operation. And yet she is one of the most vibrant, life-embracing women I know. Yes, she has her bad days, but we all do. Yes, her pain has been extreme, but so has others'. Yes, it sucks that she's ended up in this condition, but she feels it's made her a stronger, more empathetic person. She's a talented writer and I fully expect to see her work on the shelves in a few years.

This couldn't happen if Sue let society's view of her condition rule her thoughts about herself and her life. She's taken what she has been dealt and is playing it to the fullest. So many people I've met who are fully functional, who have few or no health problems, are the ones who whine the most. We can control life to a point, and then we have to take what we've been given and make the most out of it. That's all anyone can do, and that's everything one should do.

CHAPTER EIGHT

Marathon Woman

We swing ungirded hips,
And lightened are our eyes,
The rain is on our lips,
We do not run for prize.
> —Charles Hamilton Sorely, "The Song of the Ungirt Runners"

In a marathon and even on those long distance walks I feel so free, so
myself. I mean you are out there looking ridiculous—or at least I am
in those squeeze-your-butt shorts and a floral sun visor—and there is
something freeing in it all. You sweat. Water spills down your shirt as
you slurp. And people smile and approach you…treat you like you are
the guest of honor at some fine event. You feel so stripped down in a
way—there's nothing but the route, the time, and if you will do it…
a wonderful freedom.
> —Shirley, during one of our many online discussions

When I first met Shirley (not her real name) over the Internet, we somehow gravitated toward one another, and within a few months had become good friends. Over the past couple of years, we've corresponded, talked through ICQ or e-mail almost on a daily basis, talked on the phone, exchanged gifts and tokens of friendship, and I've come to deeply value my connection with her.

The first year, when she told me she was training for a marathon in December of 1998, I grew dejected. "Oh no!" A secret jockette…what must she think of me? I'm not an athlete at all. And then one day, when I approached the subject, I found out a few things. Shirley was no jockette, no beach bunny in a thong parading around the gym. She wasn't tall and slender, with flowing, long, floral dresses the way I first imagined her. She was a very real woman, lovely, gracious, and kind, with eyes as bright and warm as any I've seen. However, Shirley is also considered large by society. She wears a size sixteen or larger, she's in her mid-forties, and she reminds me of an ageless, spirited adventurer. The wonderful thing is that she doesn't realize just how inspiring she can be—and I always try to remind her of that.

When she told me why she was doing the marathon, I realized it wasn't a competition to her. She was going to walk 26.2 miles in Hawaii to raise money for leukemia research. I knew then I wanted to interview her for this book. As a larger woman in today's society, she was facing the same hurdles women like us face every day: "You're too fat to walk a marathon." Second, she was facing her own inner demons about such a long marathon. And third, the marathon was becoming a spiritual pursuit for her.

INTERVIEW WITH SHIRLEY

Yasmine: How would you describe your attitude toward movement and your body before you decided to enter this marathon? Would you have classified yourself as an athletic person?

Shirley: I've never been an athletic person. I have struggled with my weight to varying degrees ever since childhood. I tend to find friends of all body sizes whose physical activity was limited to occasional strolls, a weekend or vacation hike, or a moderate bit of biking.

Movement, though, seemed different. I have loved dancing all my life and can't sit still when live music is playing. I've always been comfortable in water. I feel both music and water offer me something spiritual.

Yasmine: What made you decide to do a marathon?

Shirley: Walking a marathon was never anything I considered. In fact, I found it puzzling why people pushed themselves so hard. What possible good could come from running or walking 26.2 miles? Why would people want to do that unless they were competitive athletes? I never understood any of the motivations or felt any stirrings within me that this is something I would ever do.

I was walking with a friend one night when she invited me to join her to train for a marathon. I was stunned. I stammered and gave her a number of excuses, but she met every one of them with a shrug of her shoulders and answered, "Me, too." Having failed to convince her that it was an impossible task, I agreed to try. I figured I could always quit. I have a strong commitment to health care, so doing a marathon to raise funds for charity was very appealing.

Yasmine: Once you made the decision, did you fear you wouldn't be able to complete the training and actual run/walk? Did you ever consider quitting or giving up before you got there?

Shirley: I had plenty of fears, the biggest being that I had gotten in over my head. People repeatedly told me how they had done marathons. Some started in their fifties. Some with major health problems completed marathons. Some started running, but finished walking. And some walked for 10 hours to get to the finish line.

While I appreciated these stories, I remained scared. During the training, we had a coach once a week. In addition to giving us tips about warming up, shoes, and nutrition, he put us through a number of drills designed to build our stamina and speed. One night very early into the training while most of us were standing breathless and grateful for a bit of rest, he asked, "How many of you are thinking you can't do a marathon because tonight is so hard?"

Many of us were silently scraping our shoes in the dirt, but some met his eyes and nodded. "Well, forget the marathon," he said. "The marathon is not tonight. We are not doing 26.2 miles tonight. We're not even going to let that thought enter our minds. What we have is right now. It's all you know. You have this moment and the next five minutes. Your goal is not to finish a marathon, your goal is to finish this next five minutes of training. Don't go to that finish line in your head. Stay here. Stay present. This minute right now is your life. Don't lose it by thinking of what's gone and can't be changed. Don't lose it by worrying about what lies ahead."

I replayed that pep talk a thousand times in my mind as I trained. Whenever I started to get scared, I simply made the effort to stay in the present. Even though we were extending our distances each week and at the end of some weeks I was bone and body sore, I knew that all I had to do was the task in front of me. I had been able to apply the concept of living in the moment in other areas of my life, but the marathon was entirely new to me.

The training program was broken down into specific goals for each week. I did not think too much about quitting because I achieved my goals week by week. It was still incomprehensible to me, though, that I could walk 26.2 miles.

Yasmine: When you began to train, what did you do on a mental/spiritual basis?

Shirley: I made big use of what I call the tools in my spiritual toolbox. Music is one. No matter how tired I am, music never fails to lift my spirits or pace. I bought a small Walkman. Motown, the New Jersey Mass Gospel Choir, and a friend's inspirational tape kept me moving and smiling. Many, many people gave me their emotional support or contributed to help me reach the fundraising goal. So many people told me how much they admired me for making the commitment.

When I would get into a lonely place on one of the long distance walks, I would begin to remember all those people who helped me, listing their names as if they were by my side. In the spiritual sense, this was true. "Kevin is with me, John is with me, Karen is with me, Steve and John are with me, Mom is with me, Susan is with me." I'd get so absorbed I'd enter a trance-like state as I tried to recall all their names. One or two miles would fly by as my heart filled with the thoughts of these dear people who wanted the best for me.

Yasmine: What kept you going during your training? What pushed you through?

Shirley: The most immediate thing that kept me on track was my team. Six of us were assigned to a mentor. We could train alone or with the group, but reporting to the mentor was mandatory. The group training days became the highlight of the week as we laughed, talked, and listened to each other's stories. Those friendships are unique because we shared our best and worst moments with each other.

Yasmine: Did you dream about the process? If so, do you think your dreams helped you understand your relationship to your body better?

Shirley: I don't recall ever dreaming about the event or the training. It's odd that I had no dreams (or at least cannot recall them) because I usually do have anxiety dreams right before a major event.

Yasmine: You knew the marathon was going to be in Hawaii. Did that make a difference in how you viewed the whole process?

Shirley: One of the rewards of participating in these fundraising marathons is the opportunity to go to exotic or faraway locations. The idea that the marathon was to be held in Hawaii was appealing, but not really a motivational factor. As we pushed through the miles and sent letter after letter to raise our fundraising dollars, we laughed to think how much easier it would be simply to buy a ticket for a trip to Hawaii. It wasn't until very late in the training that new fears suddenly arose about the potential heat in Hawaii and the elevation. While we trained on some hills, we began to realize that significant inclines were exhausting and consumed major reserves of energy, so we were all relieved to learn the course in Honolulu was at sea level, with the exception of a slight incline near Diamond Head.

Yasmine: Did you know you were ready? Was there a time when you looked inward and knew you could do it, knew you could finish the marathon?

Shirley: There are several types of training programs for marathons. The training which we were advised to do brought us to a level of walking twenty-two miles about three weeks prior to the event and then the training was reduced to walks of two to four miles. It seemed so strange after pushing for so long and so hard to reduce training just as the event neared. For all of us who were new to this, our anxiety began to rise. How did we know we could do twenty-six miles if we had trained only up to twenty-two? By curtailing our training so near to the date, what would happen to all the conditioning we had earned?

I had to trust my mentor and believe in her. She kept reassuring us we were ready. It did not feel that way. I honestly don't think I was fully convinced I would finish until I actually reached about mile twenty-one. At that point I realized I was tired, but that nothing short of a disaster would keep me from that finish line.

Yasmine: Over the weeks of physical conditioning, what changes did you notice in your life as a whole?

Shirley: During the training, I was happier, less stressed, more confident, and never appreciated a hot bath more. I noticed that I began to think of my body in a new way. I never had realized how intimidated I felt around people much thinner than me. I also realized I was a larger, slower person in a field of fast, lean athletes. But the fascinating thing was that as time went by, I cared less and less about those differences because I knew I had earned my place by showing up and doing what did not seem probable to me or most likely to them. I also began to gain great satisfaction in watching people's mouths drop as they learned I was preparing to do a marathon. It was pure fun to watch my own concept of self being rewritten and to break down stereotypes about what large people can and cannot do.

Yasmine: Talk to me about the lead time to the actual marathon. What spiritual preparations did you make? Or did you just know that you were ready?

Shirley: About two weeks prior to the event, our coach started telling us that it was time to "kick back." After weeks of increasing distance, stamina, and trying to push ourselves, we could not believe our ears. She advised us not to do more than a total of forty-five minutes walking each day and to concentrate on keeping life stress-free. It seemed so odd. "Wasn't there anything else we should do?" we asked. "Yeah, don't do anything stupid, like trying to lose a fast five to ten pounds, starting to train in new shoes, forgetting to drink water, deciding to party and consuming alcohol, eating new foods a few days prior to the event. Do what has worked before and make no changes now."

Many friends came forward during the last two weeks with small notes and gifts. One friend gave me a copy of the story *The Little Engine That Could*. Others let me know that no matter what happened on the day of the event that I had already won by simply accepting such a big personal challenge. I let all of that energy and love soak in and tried to let it steep into my memories and cells, knowing I'd need all of it to finish those 26.2 miles.

Yasmine: During the marathon, what occurred? You had been training for so long, you had accepted an incredibly strenuous task, and now it was actually happening. Take me through it with you.

Shirley: It was a shock to realize that since the marathon would begin at five in the morning to avoid the heat of the day, I had to be up by three in the morning in order to get dressed and get to the starting line. Upon waking, I remember feeling as though I were watching a movie of my life. Every motion felt foreign, and I was quite conscious of keeping my emotions at bay. After wolfing down some yogurt, a banana, and half a muffin, I met my training group and we walked to the starting line together. We looked around in amazement as people poured out of the hotels lining the area and filled the streets. Thirty thousand people walked to the starting line before the sun came up.

The starting gun fired and a magnificent display of fireworks heralded our start. Cheers rose from the crowd and cameras flashed. It was difficult to remember the advice of my coach: "Start slow." As the waves of people passed me, I remember feeling a rise of anxiety. Somehow I convinced myself to stop comparing myself to others and find my own pace.

Doing the marathon in Hawaii was exciting, but the intense scenery faded into the background as the miles grew in number. I found myself needing to be quite deliberate observing my surroundings. My thoughts were a mix of past and present. So many memories of the training and the advice of my coach flooded over me. I met the eyes of all the people who had come out to cheer us on. I remember trying to say thank you to everyone staffing a water station and being inspired at times by one anonymous face in the crowd whose smile spoke volumes of encouragement. I'd brought along my tapes and for a few minutes I'd play the music to lift my spirits and pace.

At mile eighteen, I remember a bit of concern because so often people get to this point where they begin to tire and slow down. With a jolt, I recalled a friend who told me to think of his good wishes at mile twenty. The next two miles went much easier and at mile twenty, I broke into a huge grin and said a silent hello and thank-you to my friend. How could he have known how important that morale boost would be?

Passing the twenty-mile mark, I began to realize only a bizarre accident would keep me from making it to the finish line. Once past mile twenty-four, I began to get excited. I was almost there and still feeling good! Tired, yes, but not numb or exhausted. No blisters. No lead legs. No dead knees.

During the last mile of the race, many people were on the sidelines cheering us on to the finish. I remember being especially touched by all the people who had finished the marathon and had returned to see the rest of us finish.

I was now down to about the last quarter mile. I wanted to burn the memories of those faces into my mind. I felt as though I were flying on the energy. The only thing left to do was cross that finish line and it would be over. I did not want it to end. I'd love for that moment to have lingered, but that is not how life works. In equal portions of joy and disbelief, I crossed the line. A young woman came forward and raised her arms to place a shell lei over my head. I bowed my head to make her task easier. As I lifted my head, our eyes met. My eyes had the sheen of tears.

Yasmine: This event was like a climax—you had been building for weeks (months) for it, and then it was over. Was there a sense of letdown, or "what next?" Or did the one time satisfy you and you could move on to a new pursuit?

Shirley: Once the marathon was over, there was an afterglow that lasted four to six weeks. Family, friends, and coworkers helped me celebrate the victory. They patiently listened to my stories, asked to see my finisher's T-shirt, and praised me for the accomplishment. In the second month following the marathon, my friend from the marathon said, "Well, we've gotten our mileage out of that!" We laughed, knowing that we'd basked in our success but that with each passing day, the accomplishment was becoming old news. My friend felt let down, a bit adrift without the constant pressure of daily and weekly exercise goals. I felt relief and relished the newfound freedom, but also knew that there was a hole to fill. I enrolled in a spring semester writing class and swore off walking for three months, whereas my friend persisted, even walking in subzero temperatures. I declined her offers to walk with her. I wanted to dance, I wanted to write, I wanted to read, I wanted to see friends, I wanted to stay home. I wanted to do anything but walk.

However, as spring approached, I yearned for fresh air again, and I finally accepted a walking date with my friend. We did two miles and my legs claimed their payment for the three months of inactivity. In every step, I could feel pain shoot up the front of my leg from my foot to my knee. I was devastated when I remembered that I'd danced after finishing twenty-six miles. When faced with this new pain, I wanted to pull back. My friend listened to my fears, encouraged me to continue, and walked slowly with me. In four weeks, the pain had subsided. I was determined to regain at least some of my stamina.

We decided to enter some of the 5K events. Then in June, we cheered on the runners and walkers in a local marathon. I watched them enviously and joyously. I would search the line for people whose spirits seemed to be sagging and call out their race number. I shouted encouragement and tried to make eye contact. We clapped our hands and shook noisemakers. In those moments, I could feel the desire rising in me. I wanted another marathon. I wanted to be among them. I wanted the feeling of pushing myself. I wanted to feel the floating sensation of being fully suspended in the moment, a humming unification of mind and body.

Yasmine: What were the lasting changes for you on both a physical and spiritual/mental level?

Shirley: Now, seven months after the marathon, I can see how it has made me more confident about taking risks in other areas of my life. I have the sense that I can take care of myself. I am more willing to walk into unknown situations. I've come to a more comfortable place with my body. Sadly enough, there are no lasting physical changes. My coach would often say, "No matter how many miles you've done and no matter what you feel now—every mile is its own mile." I've learned that to be true. I can start off feeling tired, and within three miles, feel a burst of energy and joy that makes me forget my weariness. I can be floating at mile twelve of a fifteen-mile walk and by mile fourteen I am dragging.

Yasmine: How did this experience affect your sensual self?

Shirley: I realize there have been changes in how I see myself and how much the physical activity has changed my physical and sensual self. I pamper myself more. I started using makeup for the first time.

The actual makeup is not that important—I realize that using it affirms that I care about how I look; I am feeling I am a worthwhile person; and that makeup can be a fun experience that enhances my spirit. I've let my hair grow much, much longer and am relishing a tousled head of curly hair. I find that I move differently. I do not feel apologetic for my body because although it is large, I know it is strong. Movement comes more easily and I find myself seeking dresses that swing and fabric that flows. I'm also watching with some fascination that I'm meeting the eyes of men whom I meet with a smile.

Yasmine: When you look at yourself now, knowing you finished a big task, what will you do next? And will you continue to pursue physical activity like this? Does your body crave it now?

Shirley: I don't think my body craves physical activity. I just don't think I'm geared to gravitate there. I seek out bookstores, museums, shows, coffee shops. I look at gyms, sports stores, and ski slopes as foreign territory. I am willing to visit there now, but it still feels as though I'm there by the grace of a visa; I'm not a resident of that world. I'm back into training for another marathon, but for me achieving the goal of going faster to cut my time is not as seductive as the emotional, spiritual, and mental process. Training for a marathon can be a metaphor for how one lives life. What is learned in that process gives one invaluable insights as to one's fears, character, strengths, and vulnerabilities.

Yasmine: What advice would you give those people who would like to set a goal like this for themselves, especially if they don't consider themselves particularly the athletic type?

Shirley: If people are not athletic but want to become more physically active, I'd suggest setting some time aside to determine what activity suits them. While being in a marathon seemed a strange endeavor for me to undertake, I soon recognized what elements drew my interest and helped me succeed. I enjoyed and needed the support of others. I needed a sport which allowed me to test myself, but not be competing with others. I think it helps to know what pleases you and what motivates you so that you can choose something that enhances your life rather than adding new stresses.

Yasmine: Any last thoughts on the subject?

Shirley: As a large woman, I know there are places in my life where I've held back from fully participating. In the marathon I met so many people who were also confronting their own struggles. For each of us, showing up was not easy. There is a tremendous satisfaction in simply showing up. At one of the races, a woman wore a shirt with this slogan: "I may not be the fastest. I may not be the meanest. I may not be the leanest. But I am *not* scared." The slogan empowered me. I might not be the best, I might not even make every goal I set, but I can live life in a way that defies fear.

Note: Shirley participated in the marathon again this year. It was harder and more taxing for several reasons, but once again she finished and triumphed over her fears.

CHAPTER NINE

The Divine Nature of Movement

I celebrate myself, and sing myself.

—Walt Whitman, "Song of Myself"

Since the time of the Greeks and before, athletes have been revered. Herakles, one of the greatest of them all, was the original strong man/ bodybuilder. The British Macha proved to us that a pregnant woman could outrace the fleetest horse. Physical aptitude has always had a connection with the Divine. Most of the gods have been portrayed as incredibly strong and immortal. We project our desires for physical perfection upon them and then aspire to match those visions.

While only a few deities rule over the realm of exercise and movement exclusively, there are a number of deities that embody these energies. Below is a brief list of some of the goddesses and gods of movement, along with their background and their corresponding energies that I know. Where correspondences are difficult to find, I've made suggestions which are noted by asterisks.

If you choose to invoke these deities for ritual, please do a little more research and make sure that they are the ones you truly want to invoke. Some deities have more than one side to them, and some have dark natures. You don't want to open up an energy you aren't sure about.

The power of physical ability will always be with us, whether in the swiftness of a deer, the grace and sinuous slinking of a cat, or the endurance of the tortoise.

THE DIVINE NATURE OF MOVEMENT

Deity and Origin	Description	Corresponding Energies
Atalanta: Greek Goddess	Atalanta, like Artemis, is a nature goddess who will only marry a man who can beat her in a race. She personifies the strength of women's bodies and the ability to take care of oneself.	Gems: moonstone, pearl, quartz Flowers: mugwort, hazel, banyan Animals: dog, horse, elephant Perfumes: ginseng, jasmine
Bast: Egyptian Goddess	Goddess of cats, the dance, ecstasy, and beauty, Lady Bast is often depicted as lion- or cat-headed. Her rites often included orgiastic ceremonies.	*Gems: peridot, gold, turquoise *Flowers: rose, lotus, fern Animals: cats of all kinds *Perfumes: lotus, orange, amber
Herakles: Greek God	The son of Zeus and the mortal Alcmene, Herakles was the strongest of them all. With the ability to perform incredible feats of strength, he embodies everything the Olympics have come to represent.	*Gems: turquoise, diamond *Flowers: vine, laurel, ivy Animals: lion, bull *Perfumes: musk, patchouli
Macha: Irish Goddess	An aspect of the Morrigan, this avatar represents the fleet-footed, the daring, and the swift. She outraced the quickest horse in Ireland while pregnant and died at the winning post while giving birth to twins.	*Gems: bronze, turquoise *Flowers: white rose, vine Animals: horse, raven *Perfumes: lavender, lemongrass
Maui: Polynesian God	Trickster lord and hero, Maui personifies the chaotic run of the universe. His feats are legendary. He personifies the surfer, the dancer, the carefree joy of the unencumbered.	*Gems: coral, olivine Flowers: banana, coconut, palm *Animals: fish *Perfumes: ginger, jasmine
Medhbh: Irish Goddess	The intoxicating goddess of sexuality and strength, it was said she could mate with thirty mortal men a day and still have the energy for her battles.	*Gems: garnet, ruby, citrine *Flowers: foxglove, white ginger *Animals: horse, dog, raven *Perfumes: jasmine, ylang ylang

Deity and Origin	Description	Corresponding Energies
Shakti: Hindu Goddess	Shakti dances through the universe to join with Shiva, and through her fires, lights his ability to create. Shakti and Shiva are an inseparable couple and together they dance into life the worlds and galaxies.	★Gems: turquoise, gold, garnet ★Flowers: lotus, jasmine, poppy ★Animals: peacock, swan ★Perfumes: jasmine, rose
Shiva: Hindu God	Shiva is the passive creative force of the Universe and cannot act without his union with Shakti, or Kali Ma. He is the passion of the dance, the lord of movement.	Gems: turquoise, ruby, star ruby Flowers: geranium, tiger lily Animals: ram, owl Perfumes: musk, dragon's blood
Tyr: Norse God	Norse god of war, law, and the patron of athletes, Tyr embodies virility and masculine strength.	★Gems: copper, garnet ★Flowers: oak, pepper Animals: wolf, horse ★Perfumes: dragon's blood, musk

Guided Meditation for Movement

As with all guided meditations, make sure that you properly ground and center yourself before proceeding. Always finish the meditation completely, and try to have a bite to eat afterward—protein and some fruit. You may want to tape this meditation, or you can designate one person to read it while others follow the journey. When you come to a *pause*, allow a thirty-second beat. *Extended pauses* indicate a specific amount of time.

Relax, get comfortable, and close your eyes. Take three slow, deep breaths and slowly exhale. (*pause*)

You are standing in a wide, flat meadow which stretches as far as you can see. The stars are wheeling overhead, and you can feel the Earth turning beneath your feet as it soars along in its orbit. We are on a spinning ball in the middle of space, in a galaxy whirling through the universe. (*pause*)

As you stand, arms stretched under the night sky, you can sense the world sailing in the path through which it has danced for billions of years, and you are part of that dance. (*pause*)

The stars shimmer, ageless, finite within infinity. They sparkle down to rain a trail of light across your face. From somewhere far in the distance you hear the slow beat of a drum, the low drone of a clarinet, the shaking of a maraca. Hypnotic, sinuous, intoxicating, the music sweeps through the meadow and catches you up in its spell. (*pause*)

One, two, step. One, two, step. Your feet move to the rhythm. You can feel the pulse of the beat rushing through the world, through the soil, up into the soles of your feet. It reverberates through your feet into your calves and knees. You find yourself swaying, following the ribbon of sound. (*pause*)

Slide and circle, your spine becomes the axis around which your body moves. Follow the pattern, follow the dance as Shakti calls you, as Shiva—Lord of the Dance—summons you. Let your arms become serpents, coiling, writhing, rearing back in their ancient salute. (*pause*)

The meadow fades into the sky and you are dancing in the stars. Feel the joy in your body as you move to the ancient dream. Feel your muscles stretch as you reach to touch the lights in the sky. Feel the fire in your pelvis awaken as the Kundalini opens its eyes. (*pause*)

There is no self-consciousness in this state. You are no longer your mortal self, you are part of the dance, part of the creation that continually destroys and creates anew. And here you may love your body, while at the same time you are far more than your mortal self could ever be. Circle the world on your toes, arch your back over the moon. Feel just how strong you are. (*extended pause—one minute*)

A gust of celestial wind rushes by and you feel the distant quaking of planets. There is a stirring in the universe. It is Shakti, dancing on fire, weaving her way through the void to awaken the force of Shiva. She is radiant and awesome. She is terrifying and brilliant. She is the mother of the gods, the ancient Creatrix, and with her dance she calls for her mate. (*pause*)

Her movements mesmerize you. You have never touched beauty until you have touched Shakti. You have never felt terror until you have felt her pass your way. She dances by on a cloud nebula, stirring the etheric storms in her wake. (*pause*)

One, two, step. One, two, step. Glide behind her, caught in the exhilaration of her quest. Let yourself flow into the rhythms of the universe, dance the dream and make it real. Reach out and connect with the Divine. The Divine encompasses all that was, all that is, all that ever will be. (*pause*)

And there on a field of starlight and moonbeams waits Shiva, prince of demons; Shiva, the destroyer; Shiva, father-consort of the world. Shakti circles him, catches him in her arms, kisses his eyes that are closed in slumber. The Lord of the Dance awakens and the Great Night begins. (*pause*)

He bows to the Queen of Fire, and reaches for her hand. Feel yourself enter their dance. Shakti withdraws, teasing, then takes his hands. With outstretched arms, they lean back, balancing each other with their weight and begin to spin. Turning, twisting, whirling, they wheel through the night; the winds from their dance shake the heavens. Fire and water, male and female, they catalyze movement, they shift stagnation, they bring an end to limbo. A battle of wills, a tender intimacy. They encompass existence with their movement and create as they destroy. Spin through the stars with them, shaken out of your apathy, your body enraptured with the Divine connection of movement to spirit. (*extended pause—one minute*)

Here is creation, here is destruction. Here is the beginning, here is the end. Here is the movement of life, and here is the stillness of the void. Within the dance of their bodies, they bring forth spirit. Feel the muscles in your body, feel the heart that pumps your blood, the lungs that keep you breathing, and know that they are part of the Divine. They are more than mere organs, more than tools. They are part of this cosmos and when you use them, tone them, keep them strong, they provide a vehicle through which you may touch the gods, through which you may join the dance of creation. (*extended long pause—one minute*).

Know that you may reach this state through mirroring the dance, by discovering the joy of movement within ritual. (*pause*)

Let yourself come to rest. Follow my voice. Ten…nine…you are slowly pulling out of trance. Eight…seven…six…you are becoming awake and aware. Five…four…you feel your thoughts quickening and stirring. Three…two…take three deep breaths and when you awaken, you will be refreshed and alert. One…now take another deep breath and open your eyes when you are ready.

- Follow the elements of this meditation physically. I wrote this to the song "Indus" by Dead Can Dance (on their *Spiritchaser* CD). Put on the music after reading through the meditation, and dance as if you were dancing with Shakti and Shiva amongst the stars.
- If you have a disability and cannot dance, you may still be able to use your arms to follow the music.
- If you feel uncomfortable because you have never danced, make sure you are alone when you try this and do your best to flow into the music. You are not on a stage here, you are not being watched. Remember—become the *dance,* not the dancer.

Part III

❧

ALTERING BODY: ALTERING SPIRIT

The act of doing this slow piercing and surrendering to the experience is a transcendent spiritual event. But people in this culture have few precedents for such an exercise in self-transformation.

—Fakir Musafar, Interview in "Modern Primitives"

CHAPTER TEN

Altered States of Body

In all societies, the man or woman who is not decorated in some way—changed from their natural state—is, in a sense, decoratively inarticulate. Body decoration is a type of language or code.
—Mary Jane Haake, Body Artist

Since time immemorial, human beings have altered their bodies to represent their spiritual journeys. We have no clear records of when this began, but tattooing, body piercing, scarification, and branding have always revolved around a central theme: paying the price of pain for the honor and the right to wear a particular symbol. This symbol may be one which marks us as part of a tribe, a culture, a religion, or it may be unique, belonging to one person and that person alone. Often it is part of a rite-of-passage ceremony. Even though these modifications make us unique as individuals, when we bear them we join a culture. Today, we call this a subculture. Occasionally referred to as "modern primitives," those of us who modify our bodies for spiritual (rather than ornamental) reasons seek to express our spirituality and our inner essence in physical form.

For some it is about reclaiming our bodies after being scarred by a disease like cancer; for others, it is about bringing to the surface those spiritual forces which lie within us and connect us to the Divine.

People use body modification to mark a rite of passage—a certain age, a certain event integral to our growth, a milestone we wish to remember.

THE ELEMENT OF CONTROL

There is a primary element in body modification we now understand—that we control our bodies because we have so little control of our outer world. We are fed rules and regulations from every side, and while some of these may be necessary in this peopled world, they hedge us in and corral us. When you add social and peer pressure, the push toward conformity becomes almost unbearable at times.

By marking our bodies, we create a badge that signals that we are unique. Most body art is in some way personalized. Of course there are the trend followers, the teenagers who will do anything just to freak out their parents, but we are not talking about them here, any more than *Vogue* addresses those women who shop at discount stores. Those who do follow trends usually don't opt for extreme body modification. They get a little thrill out of the tiny rose tattoo on their ankle or the butterfly on their butt, and that's enough. We who choose body modification for more significant reasons usually become intricately linked with the culture and the art even after we've had done what needed to be done.

This need to modify one's body is truly a drive. Often you will hear someone say, "I needed to get that tattoo," or "I kept dreaming it until I broke down and accepted it." I knew for over seven years that I would get my tattoos, but I had to wait for the right time and the right tattooist. At times I would use cosmetics to sketch out the rough design to see if it felt right, and use body paint when I went to festivals. I remember going to work one day with the faint image of a green boa coiled around my arm; the markers I had used were still visible. I saw then how oddly people reacted to the marking on my arm and got a glimpse as to what it would be like once I was truly tattooed.

Over the years my need grew stronger. Eventually I began to dream of the tattoos. Shortly after I received my first royalty check, I knew the time was right. I scheduled an appointment and spent a week in ritual before the tattooing. And then I was forever marked, forever changed.

Body modification can also include various forms of plastic and reconstructive surgery, though I'm not going to go into that here. However, people should realize that this form of modification, surgery, can be as profound a change as any spiritual enhancement. A sex change is perhaps one of the most dramatic statements about one's persona that any human can make. When a woman has breast cancer, reclaiming the breast through plastic surgery can be another life-affirming change, if she decides to go that route.

Branding and scarification are forms of bodywork that tend to frighten most people, partially because of the connections the former has with slavery, and the latter with self-mutilation caused by psychosis rather than by a decision to modify the body for spiritual purposes. Branding and scarification, like piercing and tattoos, mark the body permanently. There can be no return to the body's former state. All have been used extensively throughout tribal societies in every part of the world.

THE ELEMENT OF PAIN

The first factor is the element of pain. Most adherents to body modification for spiritual purposes welcome the pain associated with the tattoo, the piercing, the brand, or the scar. The pain serves as a reminder that we must pay for what we choose to wear. It can also be seen as a badge of courage, of stamina. We can use the pain to achieve communication with the Divine in extended rituals or in shorter bursts. We offer pain as a sacrifice to the Divine so that we earn the right to wear our chosen emblem. These are rites of passages, rituals of growth and movement.

The Mayans had extensive piercing rituals, some Native Americans the Sun Dance, the Oglala Sioux the O-Kee-Pa ceremony of hanging by flesh-hooks, the Hindus the Kavadi-bearing (or Spears of Shiva) ceremony. All of these ceremonies seek connection to the Divine through extensive pain- and ecstasy-filled rites of piercings of the skin. Modern tribalists like Fakir Musafar have reclaimed these practices and legitimated them in the West. I think it important to point out that Musafar noted that since he wasn't Native American, he did not try to recreate the Sun Dance ritual, but instead formulated a version that was appropriate for him.[1]

When we look at rituals that are extensive as some of these are, sometimes we judge them as insane, horrific, or outlandish before we examine the context and the people who are doing them. I believe that when we make judgments like this, it is as bad as judging people by their color or sex before getting to know them. There are cultures worldwide that still practice extensive rites of pain that would be outlawed in the United States. If people consent to undergo these rites, which are part of their religious heritage, how dare we judge them as wrong?

Pain is usually thought of as unpleasant. I've been in chronic pain, and there is little nobility to it other than the opportunity to learn how to master it, or to rise above it and remain true to yourself. But when someone takes pain on voluntarily to communicate with the Divine, to reach out in ecstasy to learn and understand and experience the universal flow, it is another matter entirely. When you give yourself over to the sensation rather than block or subvert it, you allow yourself to become a conduit and thereby learn how to channel the feeling through your body instead of repelling it. You not only increase your ability to withstand the minor aches and pains of daily life, you also tap into a natural source of endorphins which can trigger ecstasy.

Many of the gods required sacrifices of pain or life force. Even Yahweh demanded sacrifice of animals—and in Abraham's case, his son. Whether or not this sacrifice was aborted doesn't matter; the intent was there. Some deities have demanded human blood or flesh. Various Santeria traditions still involve animal sacrifice. In the Jewish kosher laws, the animals must be killed in a specific way in accordance with ritual. What is the difference between sacrificing a rooster during a ritual and then consuming the flesh after the Divine has feasted on the life-essence, and chopping off Henrietta Hen's head and roasting her for dinner? The only difference I can see is that the rooster received a more honorable death when his execution was an offering to the Divine. Henrietta died solely for our dining room table.

I myself would not kill any animal for sport, nor for ritual unless I intended to eat the creature. Nor do I in any way condone the torture of animals or human beings. But if people choose to undergo painful rituals voluntarily, I accept that as their right, and in many ways I understand it, for I've welcomed the pain of my own tattoos.

PREPARATION FOR A BODY MODIFICATION

First and foremost, make sure you are willing to bear this for the rest of your life! Some modifications are reversible. Sometimes a hole will close itself in time or you can have a scar removed, but for the most part anything you do to your body is permanent.

"But now you can get laser treatments to remove tattoos," you say. Yes, you can for some tattoos. The bigger pieces don't come off readily. Moreover, it's very painful and costly to remove a tattoo. Stop and think for a moment. You've marked your body in a spiritual manner—you have imprinted that energy onto your skin. What do you think removing it is going to do for you? Wipe it out as if it never existed? Not likely—any time you take on a mark that signifies a vital part of your life, you not only imprint that energy on your visible skin, but also on your aura. There's no turning back for such things. You may cover it up, you may wipe it away with a laser, but the fact is that you have accepted that energy into your life, and you will forever be changed by it. Wise up before you have the chance to regret what you are doing. Make sure this is the right course. In twenty years, will you be so sure?

I recently had bind runes for my deities tattooed on my shoulder, and a piece specific to the Dark Huntress side of Mielikki tattooed on my upper left arm. This was a major step and I would not have done it if I had not already pledged my life and soul to them for this lifetime. Essentially, I'm branded with their sigils, and I wear their energy constantly. I am theirs; there is no going back; there is no revoking this decision. If the gods don't want me, they'll kick me out. Not the other way around.

I waited for seven years between knowing I would have to get my first tattoos and actually having the work done. I've never regretted it, but they have changed me for good.

Once you know this is the right thing for you to do, you must find a good body artist. There are a number of questions you should ask. Remember, you are paying this person to alter your body permanently, and you need to trust them and know they do good work. Look through this checklist for some pointers.

- Is the body artist's shop clean and sterile? This is vital for anyone who works with needles of any sort. Do they have an autoclave in which to sterilize the instruments?

- Does the body artist work privately or will you be exposed to anyone who comes into the shop?
- Will the tattooist show you the unopened package of sterilized needles before opening it to work on you?
- Does the body artist have a portfolio of work so you can see some samples?
- Is their work of high quality? Do they belong to a professional organization?
- Does the body artist fully explain the process to you or do they seem irritable if you ask questions? My tattooist accommodates his magickal clients. I've taken ritual gear to the shop, and he approaches the art from a spiritual point of view.
- Do you click with that tattooist's energy? This is important. If you and the body artist do not mesh, you will find a lack of energy in your tattoo. Whatever energy this tattooist puts into a tattoo stays there.

Remember, you are hiring the artist for their services, and you have a right and a duty to yourself to ask these questions. You are responsible for ensuring that you have a safe and satisfying experience during your tattooing, piercing, or whatever you choose to have done. You cannot rely upon others to make sure that these conditions are fulfilled. You must go in knowing what to look for. If an artist balks at any of the above questions, leave and do not do business with them.

After you've ascertained that this person is someone you want to work with, you should ask them what they require. My tattooist will not work on people who are drunk—if you drink before a tattoo, you will bleed more and scab more, risking both an infection and a ruined tattoo. Can you smoke in the shop? Have food or drink in the shop?

Can you bring a friend to watch the work? Find out these things in advance.

If you go into a shop for a tattoo or piercing and stand there saying, "Gee, I don't know what I want," you shouldn't be there. If you go in just to browse and get ideas, but then go away and think for a while, that's a different matter.

Once you set a date and time for your modification, you can approach it in a number of ways. Most people who get tattooed or pierced probably don't think much about it beforehand. However, if you are approaching this from a spiritual point of view, it makes sense to think about how this symbol will impact your life. It also seems appropriate to view it as a rite of passage. Any time you make a significant commitment to something, any time you alter your energy in a permanent fashion, you should understand that it will change not only your aura, but also your outlook.

Perhaps this is the time when we need ritual most—when we're undergoing change, when the Wheel is turning in our lives and we aren't sure just how these alterations will affect us. Because I guarantee you, a major modification for spiritual reasons will change you, sometimes in ways you will not expect. I had little idea when I first got my tattoos just how much they would impact my life, but I did realize that I was moving forward, and so I prepared for each of them with a week's worth of ritual and focus beforehand.

At the beginning of each week before my tattoos, I laid an altar specific to the image I was getting: images of the tattoo, links to the animals, paintings of their Divine essence. I bought fresh flowers and food to celebrate the coming change in my life. Then I cast a Circle, invoked the energy that I was calling forth from and to my body.

Panther, obsidian soul who walks the night, you prowl through the branch-laced canopy of treetops. I evoke thee from my core to rise and wake, to pad fully upon my breast, to emerge from my inner core and stare through my eyes into the world. Oh, let me see with your vision, light in me the fires of your hunting spirit as I stalk the paths of my life. I call to you through ages past; we share a link as old as time. Feline Mistress of the Emerald Eyes, turn your gaze on me as I stand, unwavering. Passion prowling, feral spirit of my spirit, arise and come forth. Spirit of the Jaguar, hear me and envelop my life. I will not dishonor your essence.

Boa, emerald tree serpent, you slither through the night, passion preying. I evoke thee from the core of my Kundalini, arise and waken. Slip into my life and rest fully upon my arm. Enter my dreams and lead me on transformative journeys as I dance the paths of my life. Coil around the core of my spine and awaken my chakras to brilliant flames. Healer, destroyer, sensuous spirit of my spirit, arise and come forth. Spirit of the Boa, hear me and envelop my life. I will not dishonor your essence.

Peacock, fan your tail of one thousand all-seeing eyes. I evoke thee from the core of my spirit; arise and waken. Strut into my life and show your brilliance fully as you take your place upon my leg. Lead me into the labyrinth of language and beauty, of confidence and strength, as I stride through the paths of my life. Teach me to preen, teach me to shine. Open the doors to my psychic sight and clear my head and thoughts. All-seeing alarum, regal spirit of my spirit, arise and come forth. Spirit of the Peacock, hear me and envelop my life. I will not dishonor your essence.

I envision the tattoo as it will look, I welcome the spirit of the ink to my arm or leg or breast, to my skin. Meditation is very important to me during this week. I spend time focusing on the animal or image I'm getting, and let the spirit of the image sink in to me.

I dance my animal in trance work, evoking it from my core, for all of my totem tattoos are truly part of me before I get them—I'm just bringing them to the outer layers, rather than leaving them inside. My dreams are usually filled with visions of the spirits behind the tattoo and how they relate to me during this week. By the time I go to get the tattoo, I've come to the point where I can feel it there, and the energy is fully risen, just not inked on yet.

For my bind runes, I meditated with my deities for weeks before having them done, and it was obvious to Ray, my tattooist, how deep the energy went. He commented at one point, as he was inking the Dark Huntress tattoo, how "you must be channeling that energy directly through your heart, because it's sucking me deep."

For a piercing, scarring, or branding, I think the process is similar. Once you can see it in your mind as part of you, then your body is prepared to receive the modification. You must find a way to claim the modification as your own, and for spiritual markings there's no better way than to personalize a ritual for the coming rite of passage.

SOCIETY'S REACTIONS

While not every form of body modification is right for every person, and while some people are averse to all forms of body modification, there is a difference between offering an opinion that you don't find it appealing or even that it turns your stomach, and saying that the ritual, rite, or tradition is wrong for everyone.

Unfortunately, in our country and in cultures that have little tribal sense of belonging, we tend to run up against stereotypes all the time.

Until recently, tattoos were relegated to the realm of bikers. Beyond getting your ears pierced, piercings were for the pages of *National Geographic*. Branding? Something done to cows. Scarification? "Didn't those followers of Manson do that—cutting X's in their foreheads?"

Body modification can be viewed as erotic or offensive. Killian Li, much-tattooed and multiply-pierced, says, "I felt stronger, more myself. My social group was mostly very supportive and appreciated my reasons for doing it. Society, on the other hand, is not so appreciative."

Many people seem uncomfortable when they see my tattoos. River Willow says, "People in south Georgia are very conservative. When they see a tattoo, they think you are weird and different."

I have found this to be true even though I live in a liberal area. I've experienced everything from people stopping me to compliment me on my tattoos, to men licking their lips at me behind my husband's back, to women starting to smile, then seeing the snake on my arm and looking disgusted, to people actively wincing as they watched me walk down the street.

In a sense, these reactions allow us to pick out those people we don't want as friends. It's one thing not to appreciate what someone does with their hair or body; it's entirely different to condemn that person.

We will always form assumptions about people. This is part of human nature. However, we should be at a point in our evolution where we can go beyond this automatic process of judgment. We must learn to recognize the moment we make such snap judgments, and stop to check to see whether or not we are justified.

We must restructure our views of normality and what is acceptable. We must attempt to reach out to understand others on a deeper, less superficial level before we can understand their need for such unique personal expressions of the body and what such body expressions mean in their lives. There will always be a standard that we measure things against. However, the problems begin when we use that standard to bludgeon and berate others.

1. See *Modern Primitives*, V. Vale and Andrea Juno, p. 34.

CHAPTER ELEVEN

The Spirit of Ink

THE PAINTED PANTHER

I am home from the tattooist, aching. My leg is on fire, the pinpricks of a thousand bees still tingling. In ten minutes I can take the bandages off. It's been two hours. My third tattoo is the end of a cycle—my totem series. The first cycle of the journey that began a year before is now complete. I am a marked woman, brilliantly defined in images and colors on various parts of my body. Tattoos coil around my body; they've now become a part of my very existence. I cannot imagine life without them.

The date is May 1, 1999—Beltane. I knew eight years ago that I would bear these images. I did not know when, but my heart told me that one day I would wear them on my skin. (Shift in the rocking chair, grimace a little. My leg stings.)

When I decided to get my first tattoo, I obtained a recommendation to a new tattooist in town and went down to visit him. My first impression of the shop, Altered States, was that it was clean and airy compared to most tattoo parlors I'd wandered past or into. The energy was clear. Artwork covered the walls on both sides, vivid cartoon-like pictures known as *flash*. Flash pieces are general designs that can be tattooed whenever a customer decides she or he wants it—unlike custom tattoos which require time for the tattooist to design them from scratch.

Tables lined the walls and on them were notebooks with more artwork. Counters with jewelry for piercing stood next to the tables.

And then I noticed something I had not seen in parlors up to this point: the area where the artists were tattooing and piercing clients was cordoned off with screens. A chain prevented people from entering this work area. If they tried, the tattooists would have time to stop them. "Privacy," I thought. "They respect privacy."

Two men work in the shop. Nick is a specialist in piercing, though he also creates amazing tribal tattoos. Ray was the one I had come to see. His arms were covered with fading tattoos, most applied long ago. A ponytail trailed down his back, and he wore glasses and had a mischievous grin. When we shook hands, I felt comfortable about his touching me. That's not usual for me.

I told him who had recommended him and I laid out what I wanted: my first tattoo would be my primary totem, a black panther, on my left breast. I knew I needed other elements in the tattoo: foxglove, a green boa (my secondary totem), a peacock's feathered fan (the peacock being my third totem), a pentacle, and a fly agaric toadstool. I knew I wanted the panther staring, proud and haughty, but not grimacing or growling. I knew the boa had to be wrapped around the panther's paws, and that the foxglove should climb up my shoulder. But this was not a place where my artistic skills were coming in handy. I consulted my intuition, decided to trust Ray, left him the list and a picture of foxglove, and agreed to come back in two days to see what he'd worked up.

When I returned, I knew I had found my tattooist. He had taken the pieces I had given him, and created the visual image of my spiritual connection with Panther. Down to the color of the eyes, he had her pegged. I looked at that, looked at him, and knew that I had found the person who could see through the mists, who could etch what I felt in spirit on my body.

Twice I returned and on the third time, he did the work. Each tattoo session had a spirit, a life of its own, and each time the ink took to my skin in a different way—with the panther it sucked in, and I watched in the mirror as the dark cat came to life. My boa slithered up, painfully coiling around my arm. The peacock pierced deep, the needles carving channels on my leg in which the ink flowed with the sweep of the tail feathers.

When the panther was being done, I was afraid that I wouldn't be able to stand the pain. These are all huge pieces of work, not minor markings, and each one took over two hours. I kept thinking: two hours or more under a constant barrage of needles—will I be able to work my way through? Will I cry? To my relief, the sensation was quite sharp in some areas, but the techniques I knew to control pain allowed me to channel it.

By the time the boa came around, I wasn't as nervous—the panther had hurt, but she had grabbed hold of me and dug in quickly. I wasn't prepared for how much more the pain increases on thinner skin, nor for the exquisite sting as the needle moved over the wrist bone. But once again, my pain control bore me through. I remember thinking, as he coiled the snake around my arm, that this tattoo would not be easily hidden, and watching, amazed, as he shaded it so it looked like the boa was rearing up off my hand with its head.

And then—the peacock. I had not realized that the peacock was a symbol of Sarasvati, the Hindu goddess of language and poetry, mother of the Vedas, goddess of grace and song. I had known the peacock must have fifteen runes within the tail feathers, and those I had already decided on. I knew that it must be on my left outer calf. I had thought it should be in greens and purples, but when I got to the shop and saw the magnificent design that Ray had come up with and the colors he envisioned, I placed my trust in his art, in his sense of the piece, and let him color it. Vivid blues, purples, fuchsia—one of my favorite colors—found their way all over the bird, and a golden yellow created a kaleidoscopic vision. Though the peacock is a male bird and the tattoo is huge, stretching from my knee to my ankle, it is most decidedly feminine. Since Ray used a heavier gauge needle for the outline to make the bird stand out vividly, the pain was teeth gritting and required all my strength to channel it through.

(Shift again, and think how glad I am that I sleep on my right side so that my leg won't be touching the sheets. But the cats have to stay out of the room—can't let them chance scratching me or rubbing up against it. And pulling cat fur off a fresh tattoo hurts. And now I really do fit my nickname—the Painted Panther. I have become the vision of my soul.)

THE TATTOO

The needle was made of bone, the ink was soot and ash, charcoal powder, ground to dust and made into a paste. In an excruciating ritual, the young boy underwent a rite of passage as the shaman pierced his skin over and over, driving the ink under the epidermis. He would be marked forever as one of his tribe.

The process of tattooing has changed tremendously, and yet it still consists of using a needle to inject ink underneath the top layers of the skin, where it becomes a permanent addition to the body.

Never let anyone tell you that tattooing is always pain-free and easy. Some tattoos won't hurt too much, depending on their placement, size, and your own pain threshold. Others will feel like a stinging swarm of bees.

Every tattoo I've had has taken well over two hours, and let me tell you, having needles pierce your skin for that long is not the most comfortable experience. The places where the skin is thinnest, where there's not as much fat, or where it's right over bone hurt the worst. Ankles, hands, wrists, inner arms are rough. The one on my breast hurt least of all, interestingly enough. The one on my leg hurt the most, but we were using a heavier needle so the bold coloring would stand out more. The ones on my arm, the snake and the flowers (which were added a year after the snake was done), hurt quite a bit and bled a lot because the skin is thinner.

The first thing your tattooist will do is outline the piece. Most often, his or her design will be in washable ink on transfer paper. My tattooist shaves the area to be tattooed, then carefully places the design on my body, pressing it down hard. Once he cautiously lifts the paper, the design ink has transferred to my skin.

Next, he uses a heavier needle for the outline to make the tattoo stand out. Most tattoo guns have a series of three or five needles. You generally don't see the needles, but the gun does make a buzzing noise. However, it's not nerve-wracking like a dentist's drill. The outline hurts more than the inside of the painting. I liken it to a bee that won't let up, that continually stings you. If you are having a larger piece done, you may find that after about twenty minutes, you begin to get numb and don't feel it much.

If you are having the tattoo filled in, the tattooist switches to a different needle once the outline is done and begins the coloring process. The coloring generally goes quickly and is not as uncomfortable as the outline except on thinner skin or over bone. My boa bled like crazy because the skin on the arm is so thin.

Don't flinch. If you do, you may ruin your tattoo. Use your breath to help control the pain. Don't drink before getting a tattoo or it will bleed more and scab more. When it scabs more, chances are higher that you'll need repair work.

When your tattooist finishes, he should put a layer of petroleum jelly on your tattoo, cover it with a bandage, and send you on your way with instructions. After two hours, take the bandages off. With a moist but not dripping cloth, wash the tattoo with an antibacterial soap. Put a sparse layer of Bacitracin ointment over the whole tattoo to keep it moist, but don't clog the pores so your skin can't breathe. Don't scratch; you will ruin your tattoo. You can slap it when it itches as it's healing (this really does help). The itching can be unbelievable, but it will pass. The tattoo will flake and peel after about a week to a week-and-a-half. This is normal. Gently wash the tattoo once in the morning and once in the evening, pat it dry, and reapply ointment. Within two weeks, it should be healed up.

Don't go into the sun while your tattoo is healing. Don't soak in the tub if it will get wet. Don't do stupid things such as dropping a bit of hair developer on a relatively fresh tattoo when you are dyeing your hair. Don't spray perfume on it (yes, yes, I did, and boy did that smart). Again—if it itches, give it a sharp slap. The irritation will subside.

THE PAIN PROCESS

At one point, I talked with my tattooist about the pain process. I explained how I channel it. He said in twenty-eight years of tattooing people, he had never someone with whom the process went so quickly and smoothly, that what normally takes three hours to tattoo on most people will take two on me. He added that in all of my major pieces (which are quite intricate), he has been blown away by the way they seem to form themselves. He told me this after I mentioned that I'd been in ritual off and on all week before the tattoo. He said he could tell.

As I approach the date for my first tattoo, I realize that I don't want to fear the pain. In meditation it strikes me: the pain is a sacrifice for the right to wear these symbols of power. We don't get anything free in this world; there is always a payment or a reaction.

When I get to the shop, I sit in the chair and focus on what is being done to me. The image is clear, since I have spent hours welcoming the tattoo to my body. Ray is ready; I see the light of the artist in his eye. I take a few slow, deep breaths and nod, trying to exhale as he touches skin. Zing. The electric charge of needle on skin. Wince, but continue to breathe rhythmically, deeply.

Focus on the pain rather than on other things. Take it in, let it overwhelm me. Sink deep, keep my mind trained on the feeling of the needles as they furrow a channel along my body, as they trace a line in blood and ink. I am the canvas; Ray is the channel for the Divine. Take another deep breath, sink to a lower level, and allow the sensation to envelop me, to swallow me up. A thousand bees swarming with a single stinger.

Take this feeling, bring it inside so that we are no longer separate. No longer a blanket, the fire on my flesh becomes a lightning bolt from the spirit of the ink, etching a vision of the Divine onto my body. Take another deep breath, sink to a lower level, ride the rhythm of the needle. Feel the pain race through my body and channel it up my chakras, out my crown. Offer it as a gift to the gods. This is the price, this is my payment. I feel the streaming energy pour out of my body as I make the sacrifice.

Glance at Ray, nod as he asks if I'm okay. His eyes flash with the light of the creator. This man is married to the ink; it's in his soul.

Ten minutes in and I feel a growing sense of connection. The outline is slowly taking shape. For this piece, it will be a while before all the lines are drawn. Ease back, breathe deep, listen to the hum of the gun as it changes my skin forever. I want to feel each prick, each sting which now dances with abandon through my heart, across my soul. I woo the pain, search it out, follow the thread of ink-stained kisses that burn my body. I suck them deep, transform them into celebration and offering, release them.

"Yes, come on, that's right. Good, good, good...." Ray coaxes the design to life as he continues the outline. I don't like to talk during this time—I prefer to focus on the energy. And then, there is a shift. I feel the transition, and I start to rise on the back of the winged dragon. Rather than sinking, I now feel myself caught on the updraft as endorphins start to kick in. I soar, lean back, enjoy the rush as it spreads through me like an orgasm after a long time without sex.

I look up, smile at Ray. The pain is now channeling directly through me, I don't have to focus on it as much. I glance at the work and smile again. "Looking good," I say. He laughs and we begin to talk.

By now, I'm starting to numb up, though the pain on these large pieces never fully goes away. I'm able to talk to him more and we chat. When a spot that hurts comes along, I once again focus on channeling the pain. Over the times he's worked on me, I notice that when we talk, we tend to end up on discussions that mirror the energy of the tattoo.

Controlling pain, channeling pain, requires that you do not deny the ache, but experience it without holding onto it. Women in labor do much better if they don't fight the pain, but breathe their way through it and let go when it passes.

Breath control goes a long way toward withstanding pain, and I've used it effectively many times, from chipping my ankle bone, to the tattoos, to dental work. When we are in pain, we tend to hold our breath and to breathe in shallow pants rather than in full, deep breaths. This tenses our bodies and makes it more difficult for us to let go. We trap it in our bodies with our tension.

By learning to relax your body and breathe rhythmically with the ebb and flow of the pain, you can learn to release it. The ache becomes bearable, your body doesn't undergo as much stress, and your blood pressure will remain better.

Exercise in Breath Control for Pain

I am not going to advocate that you practice putting yourself through pain just to prepare yourself for eventual mishaps or for endeavors such as getting a tattoo. However, the next time you find yourself in mild discomfort (it's easier to start when pain is not at its highest), try this exercise. For example, let's say you have a mild ankle sprain. Take three slow, deep breaths. Let out the last one and settle into your body. Work through your muscles as you did in previous relaxation exercises in this book, slowly tensing each muscle, then letting it relax. Avoid doing this to the sore ankle. Focus on the rest of your body, breathing slowly as you go.

Now bring your attention to your sprained foot. Do not tense and relax it, as that will make it hurt more. Focus on the muscles surrounding the sore spot—the ones that are attached to the sore spot, but are not hurt themselves. Again, do not tense and relax. Simply feel the tension that you will find there—pain always brings stress to the body. Experience the tension in the muscles surrounding the trauma and slowly begin to relax these muscles in the following manner.

Take a slow, deep breath and as you do, channel that tension into your breath. Now hold your breath as you totally allow yourself to feel the tension, then slowly exhale and feel the tension flow out of your body along with your breath. Repeat this if necessary. You should notice a definite lessening of stress in the muscles surrounding your ankle.

Next, focus on the pain itself, the injured part of the body. Quite often sprains and other traumas will bring with them twinges of pain—

waves, so to speak. Wait until you feel the wave starting to build and take a slow, deep breath, focusing totally on feeling the pain—let it enter you, don't fight it, because resistance will make it hurt more.

Breathe in to the count of six or eight, then hold for a brief count and slowly exhale, and once again feel the pain whistling out of your body with your breath. Once might be enough, or you may have to do this a couple of times if the wave is long enough. After it's done, then take a couple of deep but shallower breaths through your mouth (again, as though you are in labor) to settle yourself. You'll find the pain easier to ride out this way and the breathing will keep the rest of your body from absorbing the impact.

While this will not negate the pain—it's not meant to—it will help you cope with sudden traumas and also with getting tattoos.

A CONVERSATION WITH RAY FIGUEROA, TATTOOIST

Ray Figueroa was kind enough to allow me to interview him about his work so that we might see the art form from the other side of the needle. We settled into the library's cushy chair and I set up my tape recorder.

Yasmine: Tell me a bit about yourself.

Ray: I'm forty-eight years old. I've been tattooing for twenty-eight years, almost twenty-nine. I've traveled all over the United States, as well as internationally. I've been a sign painter for thirty years and worked the truck stops pinstriping semis. I like to fish. I like the outdoors. I've been in the art field literally all my life.

Yasmine: How did you come to tattooing? What appeals to you about using skin for canvas?

Ray: It's a make-no-mistake situation. When somebody comes in with an idea, I can take that thought and make it permanent. It's like a rush, like painting a sign on a truck that's going to be driving down the freeway. Thousands of people are going to see that sign. Let me give you my story: I wasn't a very good father and didn't really see much of my children. But a number of years ago one of my daughters ran into a lady in Los Angeles. The woman had some outstanding tattoos and proceeded to tell my daughter where she had gotten them. She said the one on her leg, one of her favorites, she had received about twenty years ago from a tattooist in San Diego on Broadway. My daughter asked his name. The woman said, "Ray, or Raymond." "Figueroa?" my daughter asked, and the woman said yes. And my daughter said, "My god, that's my father." From that point on, it was something she could relate back to me. It brought her back into my life. My tattooing brought my children back. I have eight grandkids. My kids can trace my steps through all my tattoos throughout the country.

You'll always remember your tattoo artist till the day you die. And each tattoo I do, there's a bit of me going into another person. You know the idea, "pass on good thoughts, pass on good energy"? Well, if I do good work and put my soul in each piece—and I believe we have an endless amount of soul—then I'm sharing my soul with everyone I tattoo and everyone who sees those tattoos.

Yasmine: When did you first realize you had artistic talent? Have you always considered yourself an artist?

Ray: I've never considered myself an artist, but I've always created art. When I was young, we lived in a small town, a farming community, and my father owned a Greyhound bus depot. When I was around five years old, he noticed I had artistic ability. He didn't allow me take woodwork, shop, metal shop, like all the other kids. I was the one child who was given everything I needed for my art. I was allowed to paint on my bedroom walls and ceilings. My father was a great influence; he pushed me into the world of art. In fact, I took my sign painting apprenticeship at fifteen…well, at fourteen, and by fifteen was a professional sign painter. I began tattooing two years later.

I was influenced significantly by Walt Disney and of course by my father. I have a lot of relatives in the movie industry, so there are influences there as well. One of the first caricatures I drew was of Bob Hope, whom I saw on TV. We got a letter back from him saying, "Thank you very much." [laughs] You know, this was a fifteen-year-old kid's work off the television. It wasn't the greatest caricature in the world, but it was fun. But no, I've never considered myself an artist. I just happen to be in the art field and have been able to make a living off of it my entire life.

Yasmine: How did you learn the art of tattooing? What was your apprenticeship like?

Ray: I was introduced to it when I was about sixteen. There was this young fellow who had come out of prison, San Quentin to be exact, and since he had been sent there at a young age, when he came out the only people he could relate to were young teenagers. He befriended a friend of mine and me. I noticed the artwork on his arms—it was unbelievable, the most beautiful artwork I'd ever seen. So he showed us how to make machines, they were called rotary machines, and I used those for a couple years.

Then I found myself in San Diego years later on one of my road trips. On Broadway on any given payday, you'd find twenty-five hundred sailors and marines. On the off paydays—hookers and strippers. And it was a hustle in those days [laughs]. But I walked into a tattoo shop with my little machine on my hip, and this old man, Al Recine—he had been tattooing for fifty years—and William Hoss Miller, we called him Hoss, we're still friends today—owned a tattoo shop. I walked in and said, "I've never had a real tattoo, and I've been tattooing with this rotary machine for years."

When I showed them some work, Al said, "Can you draw Tweety?" And I drew Tweety. And Hoss said, "Can you put a baseball bat in his hand with a nail in it?" And I put a baseball bat in his hand with a nail in it. And Al said, "This is a tattoo machine. You will never change the needle. I will change the needle. You will never tune it up. I will tune it up. This is how deep you go. Now make me money." And for a year he sat next to me, and I never changed the needles—he changed the needles. And I never tuned it up—he tuned it up. That was my apprenticeship.

On payday, we'd each do twenty tattoos. And paydays would last three or four days, and then the strippers and hookers would come in for three or four days. So we would have a week off a month. A whole sheet of flash, we'd get five dollars for it—today I charge $100 for the same thing.

Yasmine: The first time you approached a client, were you afraid? I mean, here you are, about to mark their bodies permanently.

Ray: The first tattoo I ever gave? I wasn't afraid on my first tattoo. But with every tattoo, even today, I always think, "am I good enough that my peers are going to notice it?" The clients become secondary. Once I make that design, I've already got their soul in it, and I've already put my being into it, so the design becomes inconsequential. What matters is I have the ability to impress my peers, because that's what I want to do.

Most people don't know quality artwork, but my peers do. If you have a number of tattoos, I want them to say, "Wow, where'd you get that one?" or "Wow, who designed that?" That is the kind of reaction I'm looking for. But afraid? No, I've never been afraid of giving a tattoo.

Yasmine: Tattooing has been around since the dawn of time. Tattoos change people, permanently, and often affect their aura/energy. What are your observations on the spiritual nature of this body art form?

Ray: Boy, that's kind of tough, because everyone has their own feelings about the subject. For me, on a personal level, if I like something I'm going to get it. For others, it becomes a very spiritual situation. With some people, it can change them completely. I've seen people come in for their first tattoo so nervous and scared that they actually pass out in excitement—their endorphins kick in at that point. When you get your first tattoo and it's done correctly, it can change your whole being, your whole outlook on everything. There's an old saying in the tattoo industry, "The difference between tattooed people and non-tattooed people is, 'we don't care if you're not tattooed.'" And so you join a club.

I've worked on amputees. There's a young fellow I'm tattooing now. He's a criminal lawyer. He's also had cystic fibrosis since he was six years old, and he's thirty-one now. Every year his longevity factor goes up…except now he's starting to go downhill. I'm finishing a full-sleeve on this man, and then we're going to start on his other arm.

You can tell what a difference it's made for him. When he goes to the hospital, people around him treat him differently. They're no longer afraid of his oxygen tank, of the dark colors under his eyes. They come up and ask him about his tattoos. Every tattoo I've given him has been a welding tool, from blow torches to wrenches to jigs, realistic with a color background. Now we're going to do another kind of art form on his other arm. So yes, it can have a lot of spiritual effect.

I'll give you another example. I was in Sturgis, South Dakota, tattooing, and this lady brought in her seventeen-year-old daughter.

[The daughter] was very pretty, but she'd been in a motorcycle accident and had a six-inch scar on her hip. She refused to dress for gym. She had been a cheerleader and wouldn't go out for cheerleading. I covered the scar with a long stem rose in full color. This is the first year in five years that I haven't received a Christmas letter from her. It changed her that much. She was so excited, she became unaware of her scar.

Yasmine: I've heard a lot of women get tattoos to cover mastectomy scars, things like that.

Ray: Yes, I haven't done a mastectomy cover-up, but I've done amputees. I've covered a lot of birthing scars, a lot of scars from heart operations. You have people come in with breast implants and I've covered the scars from the implants.

Yasmine: I'm sure that over the years the nature of your clientele has changed with the times. What trends/changes/fads/movements have you noticed?

Ray: Well, for the worse—every yuppie for the past six or seven years has been getting Native American eagle feathers and so on, and they have no context for them. And the girls get *Barb Wire* since Pamela Anderson's movie. For the better, tattooing has become so mainstream that our clientele has really widened out. There was a time when your clients were either military, bikers, or street people. Now we get the suit-and-ties. I tattoo a lot of families. I get a lot of mothers bringing in daughters, and a lot of fathers bringing in sons, and they get their first tattoos together.

Yasmine: So it almost becomes something you can do together that binds the family?

Ray: Yes. I've done a lot of second-generation tattoos. I don't think I'm going to be around for the third. I recently tattooed a grandmother, a mother, and a daughter—three generations together.

Locations of tattoos have changed—a mother and a daughter, both with Chinese kanji, wanted them right on the sternum. The mother had the daughter's kanji and the daughter had the mother's kanji.

And you have to remember, I'm older than most of my clients. I've been tattooing longer than some of my clients have been alive. But I do get those forty- and fifty-year-olds. We had a lady in her late sixties get her first tattoo on her hip. It was Nefertiti. She was so excited she was running around the shop showing everyone how it looked. I had another woman come in and get a rose on her chest for her and her husband's twenty-fifth anniversary.

Yasmine: Talk a little bit about the ideal client. What attitude should he or she bring to the chair?

Ray: Boy, that's really tough. People have to connect with the tat-tooist. After the consultation, you need to pick each other's brains, you need to click together. For the creation of the perfect tattoo, you must feel comfortable with your surroundings and with your artist. Then everything else will fall in place. Without those two fac-tors, nothing is going to work. You will feel comfortable with your artist if he has the right creative ability and bedside manner. You will feel comfortable with your surroundings if it's clean, airy, wide open, and bright.

Yasmine: I noticed that made a difference for me when I came into your shop.

Ray: Yes. You have to sit down and talk to people, joke with them, get a good feel for them. This will make you feel comfortable and relaxed. When somebody gives me an idea, I get a rush. That's my ideal client—the one I get a rush with. So actually, every client is my ideal client.

Yasmine: What kind of clients make you cringe?

Ray: The ones who know everything and never had anything done at all. You get that constantly. "Well, I know because my cousin on my father's side told me that somebody told her…" and they've never been around a tattoo.

Yasmine: Have you refused to do tattoos on some people?

Ray: Yes, because of their attitude. If you have a bad attitude it's going to reflect on my work and whether it's good work or bad work, unfinished work or not, people are going to know who did that work and that's the bottom line.

Yasmine: Are there places on the body you refuse to tattoo? Why?

Ray: No. Everything's a piece of art.

Yasmine: *The Illustrated Man* by Ray Bradbury was a wonderful book, about a man illustrated with tattoos that came to life and acted out stories on his body. Have you ever worked on tattoos that just seemed to resonate with energy, with life force? If so, why do you think some work reacts like that and other pieces don't?

Ray: The ones that don't are your singular pieces…what I call floating pieces. Your, "Yes, we do Taz," flash pieces. But when somebody comes in and says to me, "I want a water dragon and a fire dragon, with no skin showing on my forearm," then that piece becomes part of me.

You know, I don't write, I don't spell very good, and I don't talk very good, but the energy I get from designing a piece is a rush and that rush is evident in how I do that work. It shows in the color mixtures, the movement of my hands. No matter whether it's a medieval piece, a cartoon piece, whether it's realistic, or anything else. When you're given the freedom to move with it, then if you're really into your work and you think more about the work than money, that's how your pieces are going to react. I've dreamt about fully finished pieces.

Yasmine: I've noticed that when you were doing my peacock I had a certain color scheme in mind, but something just clicked in. I let you do the color, and it was perfect.

Ray: Before I start the piece, my brain already sees the finished work and it's not telling my hand what to do—my hand is just doing it. I don't think, well, purple would look good next to green with some primer. Between my hand and my brain there's only one area left, and that contains my heart and soul. Everything else is oblivious. Those three are always in conjunction with each other.

When I'm working on a fun piece, if you'll look at my face you'll see me—I'm laughing, smiling, making stupid jokes. With a piece that's very moving, I become a little bit more quiet, my touch is very different. On a tribal piece, the depths the machine reaches on the skin is the same as the other types of art, but you can see the power of the piece coming from my eyes and my hands, and so on. When I'm tattooing a piece with a lot of waves or air or fire, you can tell the movement from my hands—whooshing, blasting it out so fast because time becomes irrelevant. For me that's how it works. I never see the present as I'm tattooing, I always see the beginning and the end, and it just happens.

Yasmine: What do you advise people to look for in a tattooist and a tattoo shop? What kind of questions do you wish people would ask you to show they know something about what they are getting into?

Ray: The very first thing you ask is, "How do you sterilize your equipment?" "Is everything single use?" "Individually packaged?" "Are you a member of a professional organization like the Alliance of Professional Tattooists?" "Can I see your portfolio?" Get a good feel for the studio. I personally like the private, partitioned-off sections. Notice what the rules are. Do they allow smoking, eating, animals, drinking, jerking off? Is your artist acting like a professional? An artist must act like a professional at all times.

Somebody called up on the phone the other day and said, "Do you know any woman artists?" I said, "No, why do you ask?" She said, "Because my husband doesn't want any man to see my breasts." I said, "Well, what you're going to get is somebody who's a lousy artist, if that's your only qualification." I've had eighteen-year-olds who get their first piece, and their mothers come back to get their first piece from me too.

Number one concern: sterilization—make sure everything is clean. For quality of work, ask to see their portfolio. Ask questions. If they're not going to answer your questions, get out of there—it's your health.

Yasmine: This should be standard, but it seems that not all tattoo parlors will give out good advice on taking care of a tattoo when you get it. What rules should people follow for taking care of their tattoos? What do you tell people?

Ray: Simple. You bandage it for two hours. The bandage helps your blood start coagulating. Then wash it with cool water and a mild soap like Liquid Dial. Liquid Dial is antibacterial and non-abrasive. Cover the tattoo with Bacitracin ointment. We find that [it] is a really good, top-of-the-line product. For two weeks, keep it sparingly moist—sparingly, sparingly moist. Don't overdo it. If you apply it too light, the tattoo will scab up; too heavy and it acts like Vaseline and cuts off the oxygen and the tattoo will come out in the wash. If there is any sign of redness around the edges, have your tattooist look at it. If it's getting infected, go to a doctor and get some antibiotics. But don't scratch. You can slap it or put ice cubes on it, but don't scratch.

Yasmine: Slapping it helps, I found that out.

Ray: [laughs] Yes. And never slap somebody's new tattoo unless you've had one also. You haven't earned the right.

Yasmine: What was the best tattoo you think you ever gave someone and why?

Ray: A guy in the military asked me, "What's the best place you've ever been?" I said, "The place I've just been, and the place I'm going to next." The same thing with tattoos. The last one I just did, and my next one.

Yasmine: People get addicted to tattoos, so it seems. I understand this on a personal level. The endorphins released by the pain seem to take you to a higher level of awareness. They're a real rush, actually. Do you find people really hooked on this part of the process?

Ray: Yes. Oh yeah, definitely so. It's like a good spanking, they always come back for more. [laughs] It becomes an addictive rush. People forget about the pain. Girls who are very sensitive to the needle have always come back for a second. Tattoos and potato chips. You know, that's just the way it works. I mean, you can't explain it. After your first tattoo you don't care about what people think anymore. It becomes a release, an inner release.

Yasmine: It also shows you how people react to you on the outside.

Ray: Yes. But you notice how people over the age of sixty think it's neat?

Yasmine: Yes, I've noticed that.

Ray: It's between the twenty-five to thirty-five year range that you get the sneers.

Yasmine: Speaking of pain, do you see differences in the way men and women react to getting a tattoo?

Ray: Yes. Women are more honest with pain, a lot more honest. Guys will tell you, "That doesn't hurt," and "I can take this," while you're watching the sweat fall off their foreheads. Then, they'll go to the bathroom and get all white in the face. Women deal with pain a lot easier than men do because of their honesty. Most women do better than Marines, to tell you the truth.

Yasmine: Have you ever had anybody faint in your chair?

Ray: Oh yeah, all the time. I just tell them it's because of my magnetism. [laughs] It happens when the endorphins kick in. Fainting is a common occurrence, very common. It's the idea of getting pricked with a needle—not the tattoo. People come in beforehand with second-hand knowledge like, "I was told that you go six feet under the thumbnail with bamboo rods and pour four buckets of paint in it." They already have [an idea] in their head of what to expect. Then the endorphins kick in, and the rush and the worry make their blood pressure drop, so they faint. Later, they think, "It's not supposed to be this easy!" One of the most common things I hear is, "You mean that's it? That's all?"

Yasmine: [laughs] I can tell you, mine hurt! You know, for me the pain was a price.

Ray: But you have larger pieces, quite a bit larger. And the locations are quite a bit different. You have the back of the forearm. And, for example, tell me the difference in how it felt between the curvature of your breast and the upper part of your breast. The upper part of your breast was a lot more painful, correct?

Yasmine: Yeah, yeah it was. And my shoulders are going to be painful, I imagine.

Ray: Right. And again, the back of your forearm was more painful than the front, correct?

Yasmine: Yes, and down near my ankle, on the peacock, hurt, especially.

Ray: Tattooing is like acupuncture. We have nerve endings all over our body. We never know what's going to hurt. Also weight has a lot to do with it, state of mind, location of tattoos—ribcage, under the arm, back of the knees are all extremely sensitive areas. So all of those are factors. Like I said, it depends on how big of a piece it is. Once that outline is done, though, the shading and coloring are nothing.

Yasmine: I have to say, that for me, the pain is a price I'm glad I pay—because for me it is a spiritual thing.

Ray: Yeah, and I'll tell you, the older you get the worse it is. I'm a wimp getting tattoos.

Yasmine: How do you perceive the continuing evolution of the tattoo industry? What changes would you like to see in artwork, in technology?

Ray: There are no limitations in artwork anymore. European tattooists have shown us that with the watercolor styles they do. The German artists, with their realistic work, the Japanese with their powerful colors, and the Americans with combinations of everything. And it's only going to get better because, while the machine is technically the same since 1923–1928, the person behind the machine has evolved.

These kids today are tremendous artists, but if they don't get taught by the old school, they're not going to get the same rush doing the tattoo, the same emotion doing the tattoo. That emotion is transferred into that tattoo and the individual wears that emotion throughout the rest of his or her life. When you give a tattoo, you have to think ten years in advance. How is the skin going to change? How is the pigment going to change? Our pigment today is phenomenal…it's much better than it was ten years ago, twenty years ago. I think it's only going to get better.

Yasmine: Is there anything else you'd like to add to this interview?

Ray: Not really, just that you want to keep it clean, keep it safe. When you go to look for an artist come to me, and forget everyone else [laughs]. Sterilization—that's your number one concern. Feel good with your artist, and remember, I have warm hands. That's about it.

Yasmine: Thanks, Ray. You're a sweetheart.

Ray: I know.

CHAPTER TWELVE

The Edge of Extreme

There are many paths up the mountain,
but the view at the top is the same.
                                    —Ram Dass

Within the realms of permanent body modification, there are vast opportunities for the individual to reach for the Divine. Three of the most common, besides tattooing, are body piercing, branding, and scarification. All three, with perhaps the exception of some forms of piercing, prompt immediate and emotional reactions from people.

Branding brings up specters of the days of slavery when people were branded like cattle. Reactions to scarification bring up fears about self-mutilation. Even some forms of piercing make us wince and turn away. However, the fact remains that these practices have been used worldwide in pursuit of the Divine for thousands of years.

BODY PIERCING

Body piercing is the act of putting a hole through the flesh into which we insert jewelry or other objects. Piercing is extremely common at this point in time and just about any body part you can name has been pierced by somebody somewhere. While a fad for many, for some it represents a tribal sense of connection with deity, with other people, and with the self. When you look at the psychic ramifications of body piercing, it's not just the act of piercing that takes on a spiritual significance or depth. Fakir Musafar makes a very good point that when we put holes in our body, we are creating psychic portals into which energy may enter.[1] Therefore, if you choose piercing with any sense of spirituality, you must be prepared to invoke the appropriate energy into your ritual to "fill up" the void opened when the flesh is pierced.

When we approach piercing in a spiritual way, we should look at what we're getting done and ask, "Why do I want this? What does this mean to me?" And we must have the answer. It's not like hopping on the bandwagon and going along for the ride. Any time we do something for a spiritual reason, we should know that we are being led to do so for our own evolution. There is no point in hoping that we will achieve the same results as someone else.

In cases like the kavadi spear ceremony of the Savite Hindus, there can be hundreds of piercings without drawing blood. This ceremony is linked with the worship and celebration of Lord Murugan during the festival of Thaipusam, during which throngs of people (not of the priest caste) make pilgrimages to various temples, as well as the Batu Caves, for the rites. Thaipusam commemorates the day Lord Shiva presented the *Nyana Vel* (golden spear) to Lord Murugan, who used it to defeat his enemies. Murugan is the child of Shiva and Parvati, and the brother of the Lord Ganesha. He rides on a peacock holding a bunch of spears.

Long ago, the *devas* (god-forms) were being attacked by the *asuras* (forces of evil). They beseeched Lord Shiva for his protection. Shiva opened his third eye and six sparks of fire flew out. These sparks of fire converged, and from that convergence Lord Murugan appeared. Shiva commanded him to defeat the asuras and gave him the Nyana Vel to do so. Lord Murugan promptly obeyed, and in commemoration of his victory, Thaipusam is celebrated. During the festival, Hindus cleanse themselves by fasting for one month, praying frequently, and abstaining from sex. On the day of Thaipusam, they will often carry kavadi.

During the evening before Thaipusam, an image of the god is showered with precious gems, then placed on a bed of flower petals. Incense is burned in his honor, and his image is drawn in a silver chariot by two bulls and devotees along a nine-mile journey from the Maha Mariamman Temple to the Batu Caves, where sacred rites are held. The celebration lasts three days.

The kavadi is an ornate steel frame that pierces the body. The devotees, deep in trance, wear the kavadi and also skewer themselves with hooks and gilt chains. No blood flows, and the worshipers seldom feel any pain. Devotees wear the kavadi in penance or to repay the gods for some service, or simply in reverence and celebration. The *kavadiyattam* is the name of the dance done while wearing the kavadi.

There are also ceremonies such as the Native American Sun Dance that use (or used—the piercing is now outlawed, though still practiced in some areas) body piercing as part of the ritual. The ceremony recreates the connection of the human spirit to Wakan Tanka, the Great Spirit. The tribes of the plains believe that through purification, sacrifice, and prayer, they become conduits for power from the Great Spirit. This ceremony strengthens the connection between all members of the tribe.

The week before the ceremony, there is a great deal of activity during which prayer and preparations take place. Often a special Sun Dance lodge is built according to complicated rituals. A sacred tree is cut for use as a center pole in the structure, and an enclosure for the dance is constructed around the tree.

As in many Native American traditions, the entrance to the lodge faces east, so that the sunrise is visible at the beginning of the ceremonies. There will be an altar inside. Those planning to dance the Sun Dance often fast during the days of dancing.

Drummers chant and drum. The dancers move back and forth from the periphery of the lodge to the center pole while continuously blowing on eagle-bone whistles, alternating periods of rest and dance. When the ceremony is finished, the dancers and drummers undergo rites of purification and then may eat and drink. The lodge is abandoned.

During the past, and even today, though it is outlawed by our government, some dancers perform acts of self-mutilation while they are in a trance state. They are pierced through the chest and shoulder muscles with skewers and hooks, and then tied to the center pole. The dancers then dance, in trance, until their flesh tears and releases them.

The Sun Dance was often performed for the good of the tribe, rather than the good of the individual. Often if the tribe needed food, they would dance the Sun Dance, asking to be shown where the buffalo were. During the trance, they would see where to hunt.

We can look at the crucifixion of Jesus and see the significance of piercing. While some may argue that he did not choose this, we might answer, "But his God chose it for him and he accepted it." Therefore, it was a religious rite that led to his death, a piercing and scarification that is viewed today as a symbol of sacrifice by millions.

If you go to Malaysia or some parts of India, you can still take part in the kavadi ceremony as it is traditionally practiced. Though I am really not attracted to most of the piercing rituals and ceremonies, for some reason the kavadi speaks to me. Whether I shall ever attempt it I can't say for sure. However, it seems to me to be one of the most intense rituals that I've read about. The Hindu deities watch the ritual; the energy of a half-million people together celebrating Thaipusam has to be a river of energy connected directly to the world of the gods. In my research on the kavadi, I've come across pictures with radiant lines of light shining across the participants that could not be explained by the photographers. I've seen the face of bliss on those who carry kavadi.

If you choose to participate in one of these rituals, make sure you find an experienced guide—preferably someone who has some medical training as well. The purpose of this is to connect with the Divine, not simply to mutilate the self. There's a vast difference between undergoing rites of pain for the gods, and undergoing them for the thrill of it.

Permanent body piercings have religious significance to many people. Perhaps they mark a significant passage in daily life. My friend Killian Li got her belly button pierced when she was sterilized to mark the reclaiming of her life from the fear of unwanted pregnancy. Another friend, Youngtree, uses piercings to "cycle energy and permanently activate specific dynamic circuits" in his body.

Commonly Pierced Areas of the Body

Nipple rings go back to ancient Rome, where the centurions wore them as a sign of their bravery and virility. Piercings are used more for adornment and sexual stimulation than in ritual, but some people use them to mark significant passages in their lives, and therefore they become ritually and spiritually significant.

Various forms of body piercing include the following:

Ampallang. Most common in areas near the Indian Ocean. The stud is inserted horizontally through the head of the penis, circumventing the urethra.

Apadravya. Found in the Kama Sutra, this Hindu piercing is a vertical piercing through the shaft of the penis, just behind the head. Once in a while the stud goes through the head of the penis.

Clitoris. Difficult to do on women with small clitorises, the ring or stud goes directly through the clitoris.

Dydoe. A piercing through both sides of the upper rim of the glans.

Ears. Used for earrings and adornment, for the most part. Piercing may be done anywhere on the ear nowadays, and multiple piercings are commonplace.

Foreskin. Piercing through the foreskin at the top of the penis.

Frenum. A ring is placed around the penis and the piercing is done through the loose skin underneath.

Guiche. Common in the South Pacific, this piercing is placed in the ridge of skin between the anus and scrotum.

Hafada. This piercing is through the scrotum.

Labia. The piercing is through the wall of the labia. Sometimes multiple rings are added to create an almost chain-like effect.

Navel. A piercing through the belly button. This type of piercing is often one of the hardest to heal correctly.

Nipple. There are several ways the nipple can be pierced, but the most common is a ring or stud parallel to the body, through the nipple.

You should go to a professional piercer for any of these—some piercings are more dangerous than others and need a trained artist, and still other piercings really need to be placed symmetrically or they will look lopsided and catch on your clothing.

Almost all of the above methods, except the ear and navel, are reputed to heighten sexual sensation to an incredible degree. While additional sexual stimulation is wonderful, it is not enough for me to consider piercing other parts of my body, although I love my pierced ears and have two holes in each ear (tame by today's considerations). I would have to be led by the Spirit to know that this was important for me to do.

There are more extreme forms of piercing—penile implants, where the penis is studded with tiny ball bearings (much like BBs) under the skin; piercings on the back for the insertion of chains, etc. However, many of these have potentially damaging side effects. I would caution you to make sure you know what you are doing before you plunge into anything, and ask yourself "why am I doing this" several times before you go through with extreme piercing.

You should follow the same basic rules for choosing a professional piercer as you would in choosing a tattoo artist and studio. Remember, piercing is a form, in a sense, of acupuncture, and you will indeed activate energy channels on your body when you have a hole placed in your skin. Often, when body piercing is done in ritual and trance, the needle will, when pressed against the skin, just slide right through without any resistance.

BRANDING AND SCARIFICATION

Branding—searing and burning the flesh to leave a permanent mark— and scarification—using cuts to leave scars in a marked pattern—are two other forms of body modification now being revived among some hardcore body modifiers.

Scarification may have had more than a spiritual basis originally. It was thought by native cultures who practiced it that by creating a series of small wounds from which your body could rapidly heal, your immune system would be more apt to kick in faster if you became seriously wounded.

Puberty rites and other rites of passage sometimes included scarification in various cultures, including tribes in the Upper Volta, Nigeria, Chad, and the Sudan. The ability to withstand pain, the ability to face the knife, marks an adolescent as brave enough to take on everyday pursuits. In some tribal cultures it was vital to know whom you could rely on in times of need and trouble, and rites of passage were one way of showing that a person had the courage necessary to take on the responsibility of the adult world. Far from being the self-mutilation or self-destruction of some of today's youth, scarification rites were a badge of honor. The scarification was not caused by psychological distress, but performed intentionally as a way for the adolescent to form a link to the tribe and its culture.

A significant proportion of modern scarification tends to be done by the individual using razor blades. However, some body artists are beginning to use scarification rather than tattoos. It's becoming a ritualistic art form. Once again, if you choose to go this route, please find a reputable body artist so that you don't end up with an infection or with the danger of cutting through a critical vein or injuring a tendon. These are all real dangers, and you must know what you are doing.

Youngtree uses scarification for magickal sigils on his body. He says, "The first were bind runes of reconciliation on both my left and right forearms. The second was a bind rune of the purest manifestation of male sexuality on my belly, below the navel. The third was a bind rune of the joyous satisfaction of Queer Spirit Brother Love on my belly, above the navel." He was also branded with two crescent moons, one on either side of his vaccination scar on his upper left arm, turning the scar into the symbol of the Triple Goddess—the Maiden, Mother, Crone rune.

Of the branding, he says, "The brandings are from a shamanic dreaming session, and are a personal dedication to a specific goddess. I have found that I am a manifestation of the meaning of each of these things that the chosen body modifications represent. I live in and own my body and yet am not my body. These processes have led me to living a direct, personal experience of the Divine. Even people who are not aware of these processes notice my transformation and are frequently drawn to me for their own reasons."

Youngtree is a fascinating man. I met him in 1992, and was immediately drawn by the intensity with which he lives the spiritual side of his life and still interacts in the mundane world. His brandings, scarifications, piercings, and tattoos have always fascinated me—they never seem done for shock value, but for true spiritual reasons. He is a dear friend, and one of those people who I truly feel crosses the barriers between gay and straight, between spirit and daily life. He simply *is*.

Branding conjures up visions of slavery and is very controversial, but what is a tattoo, if not a brand? Branding uses heat; scarification uses cutting; tattoos use ink and needle, but all have the same end result: they mark the body permanently. Remember that a brand comes out wider and bigger than the metal used to make it—if you use too large a metal brand, you will end up with a huge scar on your skin that might not resemble the original design. And certain types of branding equipment designed for, say, bovine flesh, are not suitable for human skin. Again, don't just rely on what someone says—make sure you see examples of your artist's work and you feel comfortable with that person.

You might remember the *Kung Fu* television show, from years back. One of my favorite scenes was in the opening credits, where the hero had gained enough wisdom and therefore was marked with the signs of the tiger and the dragon. I remember sitting there as a young girl watching him press his arms to the side of the hot iron box to carry it into the snow where he fainted, and thinking: I want symbols on my body. I want to be marked with the sign that means I'm part of something mystical. I chose to go with tattoos, but I remember the passion I felt when I watched the designs form on his arms, and how important and symbolic it seemed to me.

Perhaps it is the bloodletting in scarification and the flesh singeing in branding that freak out people who might not blink an eye at a tattoo. After all, with today's AIDS-conscious society, blood has become even more feared than before. There's a pervasive sense that open wounds potentially put others at risk. Even if you are not infected, no one else but yourself and your doctor can know the truth with certainty.

Therefore, it's perhaps understandable why some people might fear these forms of body modification.

I remember at a Pagan festival years ago I was with a group of friends, one of whom is HIV-positive. He cut his finger and it was bleeding. A couple of us automatically moved forward to help, but he stepped back and said, "Stay back while I take care of this." It hit me then—his blood could truly be a potential killer. And that saddened me, because I knew that he was protecting us, and I wanted to help, yet couldn't because I didn't have any rubber gloves.

I am wondering what direction society will take about this in the future. Young kids seem to be ignoring the risks of AIDS more and more. Studies show that the issue has been stressed so much that they're tired of hearing and thinking about it. We are, as a nation, longing for something deeper. We long to go into the depths of the spirit and discover a cultural unity. Yet in the United States, this is not possible because we come from so many different cultures. So we create subcultures within which to bond. Our beliefs may be different, but we connect on some essential levels that give us a sense of belonging. And one of the common facets of the subculture is marking the body for spiritual reasons.

I believe that there's a sense of emptiness in our country caused by the lack of rituals for transitional times, and therefore many people who seek this connection are creating a new paradigm for existence. Although many people will be alienated by body art, as Ray Figueroa said in his interview, tattooing is becoming more mainstream, almost a family affair. We are beginning to see a shift in consciousness about all forms of body art.

---

1. Interview with Fakir Musafar: http://www.bme.freeq.com/fakir2.htm

CHAPTER THIRTEEN

The Divine Nature
of Body Modification

We are the birds of the same nest,
We may wear different skins,
We may speak different languages,
We may believe in different religions,
We may belong to different cultures,
Yet we share the same home—our Earth.

—Atharva Veda

It is almost impossible, without undertaking a major study of the subject, to come up with a list of deities specific to body modification. Of
course we have Shiva and Lord Murugan, to whom the kavadi is sacred,
but the truth is that body art and modification have been practiced by
almost every culture, especially among the aboriginal tribes throughout
the South Pacific, Central America, South America, and North
America—it's a worldwide phenomena. Cultures like those of the Celts
and the Picts also used body art and modification. I suggest that you
meditate on any potential body modification to see if it's something
that is spiritually compatible with your spirits, deities, and your own
higher self, and then use your common sense as a guide.

As always, if you choose to invoke any deities for ritual, please research them to make sure that they are the ones you truly want to invoke.

GUIDED MEDITATION FOR BODY MODIFICATION

As with all guided meditations, make sure that you properly ground and center yourself before proceeding. Always include the last part of the meditation, and try to eat some protein and fruit afterward. You may want to tape record this meditation or designate someone to read it. When a pause is marked, allow a thirty-second beat. When an extended pause is noted, the length of the pause is specified.

Relax, get comfortable, and close your eyes. Take three slow, deep breaths and slowly exhale. (*pause*)

Focus on my words as you sit quietly. Follow their pattern, feel the rhythm, play with the dance of language as it creates pictures and images in your mind. Let yourself drift into this trance, slide into the void, dive into the abyss. Clear your mind of all thoughts except what you are hearing. Focus on the patterns built by the words. Sounds become words become visions. Visions become the dreamtime of your soul. (*pause*)

Now listen to the beat of your heart. Listen to the rhythm of your pulse. Feel your breath as your chest rises and falls. Breath beats an even rhythm. Breath twists and flows to the cadence of your life. (*pause*)

Be in your body. Take a deep breath and slowly exhale. As you exhale, feel your skin as it surrounds your body. Reach out with your hand and gently rub your other arm. What does your flesh feel like? Is it untouched—blank, a canvas waiting? Or is your skin painted, textured—does your body tell stories in pictures or scars? (*pause*)

Perhaps the thought of getting a tattoo or piercing has never entered your mind. Or perhaps you embrace the idea. Perhaps you have already undergone such a rite. For now, let your mind dwell on the possibility. What do you think of when you think of tattoos and piercings? How do you relate the thought to your own life? Does it repulse you? Frighten you? Intrigue you? (*pause*)

What do you think you would be like if you were tattooed, or pierced? What do you think it would do to your outlook, your life? If you have both, think about how they have changed you, what differences you have noticed because of them. (*extended pause—one minute*)

Listen to your heartbeat. Listen to my words. Follow the pattern, follow the rhythm. All life has a cadence. It might be swirling like a great wind, or staccato and clipped. Feel the pattern of your soul—what does it look like? What does this pattern present itself as? Take a deep breath and let yourself slide into trance as you experience the rhythm that is uniquely yours. (*extended pause—one minute*)

Now see this pattern rise to the top of your skin. If the rhythm of your soul took on form and picture, took on essence, what would it look like? What would be the expression of your being? Would it be a vivid flash of color in the shape of a coiling dragon? Would it be a series of raised scars in a tribal pattern? Would it be an ornate ring circling your nipple, runes etched on the silver? Let the pattern of yourself emerge in your thoughts. Let it express itself. (*extended pause—one minute*)

Imagine wearing the expression of your spirituality on your skin. What would it be? If you already do, how does this affect your connection with the Divine? What patterns signify your connection with Spirit? What images link you to the gods, with the Elements, with the world of magick? Take a moment to explore what your bond with the Divine looks like put to your skin. (*extended pause—two minutes*)

Turn your attention to those who go to extremes in order to pay reverence to their gods. You see a man with a steel frame around his waist. It looks like a peacock tail, spread in a half-circle. There are needle-sharp spears laced through the frame like spokes on a wheel, and they meet near his chest where the tips pierce his flesh. You see no blood and on his face is a look of bliss. He is carrying kavadi, the spears of Shiva for Lord Murugan. (*pause*)

Do you find this sight revolting? Or captivating? Would you be willing to undergo such extreme sacrifice for your gods? What would you do, on a physical level, for the deities you work with? Very few people will ever go to this extreme, but it is good to examine your reactions to such a display of reverence and willingness to give of the self for the Divine. Those who fast for Ramadan, those who sacrifice for Lent, are all making bodily sacrifices for their gods, for their beliefs. This is simply another way of showing a connection to the Divine. Can you look at this man now and see the beauty of what he is doing? (*extended pause—one minute*)

Perhaps you will never get a tattoo or piercing or scarification. These forms of expression are not for everyone. But when you can see the beauty in them, when you can see the reason behind them, you will have an understanding of another form of reverence for spirit through body.

Now let yourself come to rest. Follow my voice. Ten…nine…you are slowly pulling out of trance. Eight…seven…six…you are becoming awake and aware. Five…four…you feel your thoughts quickening and stirring. Three…two…take three deep breaths and when you awaken, you will be refreshed and alert. One…now take another deep breath and open your eyes when you are ready.

Suggested Exercises for Body Modification Meditation

- Even if you are not interested in getting a body modification for yourself, plan a trip to a nearby tattoo parlor. If it seems to be clean, light, and airy, go in and look at the artwork on the walls. See if you can extend your comfort zone about the kind of people who get tattoos.

- Should you decide to get a tattoo, do the research. Make sure you are getting what you need and the shop and artist make you comfortable.

- Perhaps you would like to explore body modification in a non-permanent manner through body painting. This is a way to explore how different it can feel to mark your body. Sometimes it can lead to either the knowledge that you are not meant for body modification, or the knowledge that you must explore it further.

- Think about how you react to tattooed and pierced people. Do they make you uncomfortable? Do you make assumptions about what kind of people they are before you know them? Examine any prejudices that you might have and see if you can find a way to negate them.

- Explore the history of tattoos or piercings on an in-depth level. See how, until the modern era in our culture, a tattooed body was far more common than a body without tattoos. Study the ceremonies of the kavadi and the Sun Dance, and learn why these were and are done.

A Long Journey, Half Complete

Daydreaming had started me on the way; but story writing once I was truly in its grip, took me and shook me awake.

—Eudora Welty

And so once again I come to the end of another book, and yet it is not an end. This is the first part in my body-spirit series and *Sexual Ecstasy and the Divine* will be coming next, which focuses on melding spirit with sexuality. Having finished this book and also having completed a good share of *Sexual Ecstasy and the Divine*, I have to say that writing these books has taught me so much—about sexuality, about people, but most of all, about myself. Each book I write leads me on a merry chase, the last few more so than any others. *Tarot Journeys*[1] led me on a journey of transformation; each meditation took me into my core and out again. *Crafting the Body Divine* and *Sexual Ecstasy and the Divine* are leading me on yet another type of journey, this time into the core of my sexuality. These books are an exposition of self, and in truth, I have offered, and will be offering, you glimpses into my own being in a way I'm still not sure I feel totally comfortable with. But this whole subject of body and spirit had been screaming at me for long enough that I knew I had to shake the concepts loose from the ether and manifest them into a form that will reach out to help others. It is my hope that this book has helped you in some fashion and that you will find equal value in its sister book.

I have been explicit and I have been graphic. I have been poetic and I have been personal. Above all, I've been open about myself and honest with you, because I want you to be honest with yourself. I want you to question your views on your self-esteem, on your body, on your spiritual connection to your physical self, on how you view others.

We are here to experience life in a temporal form; we are in-body to experience the body. We can connect our spirit and our physical selves in ways that are ecstatic and joyous. I began this book with a quote from a song I love—"I am just a holy instrument of joy."[2] I believe this, to the core of my heart: we are creatures of love and passion, of experience and joy.

Our life in this world is to be lived with enthusiasm. Of course we're going to feel hurt, pain, sorrow. We have no other choice if we are to balance out our existence. But how sad it would be if we were so numb so that neither happiness nor pain affected us. And how fitting that our relationship with ourselves encompasses both our light and shadow selves, for we are such a blend that if we try to separate the yin/yang, fire/water, we risk losing our holistic sense of balance.

When we approach the gods, we approach them not as nebulous energy beings, but as mortal, fallible as they are fallible, emotional as they are emotional. We mirror our deities even as they mirror us. We approach them through our passion, our sensuality, and our ecstasy, and in doing so, discover the Divine within our own hearts.

Bright Blessings, and I wish you ecstatic joy in your life.

—the Painted Panther
Yasmine Galenorn

1. *Tarot Journeys*, by Yasmine Galenorn, Llewellyn Worldwide, 1999.
2. "Big Fun," by Shriekback; Go Bang (Island Records, Inc., 1988).

APPENDICES
AND
REFERENCES

Magickal Rites and Elemental Charts

CASTING CIRCLES AND INVOKING THE ELEMENTS

I fully cover casting a Circle (an area of sacred space) in my book, *Embracing the Moon*,[1] so I will just discuss the rudimentary concepts here.

The idea behind casting a Circle is to create sacred space in which to practice your magickal workings. When you cast a Circle, you create a space charged with magick that is conducive to spellcraft and ritual. There are many ways to cast a Circle; you should experiment in order to find which way works best for you. You might find that you vary the way you cast your Circle each time you enter ritual. It is a good idea to clean your physical space before you enter into magickal practice: sweep, clear out cobwebs, clean up clutter. This will help prevent too much chaotic magick from filtering into your space.

The simplest and most common method of casting a Circle utilizes a wand, an athame, a crystal, or your hand to direct energy. Stand in the center of the room and ground yourself. Raise energy through your body and focus it into your hand or into the tool. Channel it out of the tool to create a line of directed force as you slowly turn in a circle, keeping your concentration focused.

You can add chants, you can create an invocation, you can cast the Circle in silence. I usually cast my Circles thrice: once in the name of the Young Lord and the Maiden, once in the name of the Father and the Mother, and once in the name of the Sage and the Crone. When you open the Circle, you can use a broom or your hand to sweep the energy away.

Invoking the Elements

Most Witches and Pagans invoke the four Elements after they cast the Circle. Together, these Elements—Earth, Air, Fire, and Water—create balance and together comprise all life. When we invoke Earth, we invoke the essence of stability, manifestation, abundance, solidity, prosperity, the physical realm. With Air, we invoke intellect, insight, clarity, new beginnings. Fire brings us transformation, healing, passion, creativity, sensuality. With Water, we find emotion, the hidden depths of the psyche, introspection, and the ability to adapt.

ELEMENTAL CORRESPONDENCE TABLES

THE ELEMENT OF AIR

Sabbats	Imbolc, Ostara
Direction	East
Realms Ruled Over	The mind, all mental, intellectual, and some psychic work; knowledge; abstract thought; theory; mountaintops; prairies open to the wind; wind; breath; clouds; vapor and mist; storms; purification; removal of stagnation; new beginnings; change
Time	Dawn
Season	Spring
Colors	White, yellow, lavender, pale blue, gray
Zodiac	Gemini, Libra, Aquarius
Tools	Censer, incense, athame, sword
Oils	Frankincense, violet, lavender, lemon, rosemary
Faeries	Sylphs
Animals	All birds
Goddesses	Aradia, Arianrhod, Nuit, Urania, Athena
Gods	Mercury, Hermes, Shu, Thoth, Khephera

THE ELEMENT OF FIRE

Sabbats	Beltane, Litha
Direction	South
Realms Ruled Over	Creativity; passion; energy; blood; healing; destruction; temper; faerie fire, phosphorescence, and will-o'-the-wisps volcanoes; flame; lava; bonfires; deserts; sun
Time	Noon
Season	Summer
Colors	Red, orange, gold, crimson, peridot, white
Zodiac	Leo, Aries, Sagittarius
Tools	Wand, candle
Oils	Lime, orange, neroli, citronella
Faeries	Flame dancers, phoenix
Animals	Salamander, snake, lizard
Goddesses	Pele, Freyja, Vesta, Hestia, Brighid
Gods	Vulcan, Horus, Ra, Agni, Hephaestus

THE ELEMENT OF WATER

Sabbats	Lughnasadh, Mabon
Direction	West
Realms Ruled Over	Emotions; feelings; love; sorrow; intuition; the subconscious and unconscious minds; the womb; fertility; menstruation; cleansing; purification; oceans; lakes; tide pools; rain; springs; and wells
Time	Afternoon
Season	Autumn
Colors	Blue, blue-gray, aquamarine, lavender, white, gray, indigo, royal purple
Zodiac	Pisces, Scorpio, Cancer
Tools	Chalice, cauldron
Oils	Lemon, lily of the valley, camphor
Faeries	Naiads, undines, sirens
Animals	All fish and marine life
Goddesses	Aphrodite, Isis, Mari, Tiamat, Vellamo, Ran, Kupala
Gods	Ahto, Osiris, Manannan, Neptune, Poseidon, Varuna

THE ELEMENT OF EARTH

Sabbats	Samhain, Yule
Direction	North
Realms Ruled Over	The body; growth; nature; sustenance; material gain; prosperity; money; death; caverns; fields; meadows; plants; trees; animals; rocks; crystals; manifestation; materialization
Time	Midnight
Season	Winter
Colors	Black, brown, green, gold, mustard
Zodiac	Capricorn, Taurus, Virgo
Tools	Pentacle
Oils	Pine, cypress, cedar, sage, vetiver
Faeries	Paras, kobolds, dwarves
Animals	All four-footed animals
Goddesses	Ceres, Demeter, Gaia, Persephone, Kore, Rhea, Epona, Cerridwen
Gods	Cernunnos, Herne, Dionysus, Marduk, Pan, Tammuz, Attis, Thor

SIMPLE CIRCLE CASTING AND INVOCATION OF THE ELEMENTS

In the center of your ritual space, stand with your dagger (or tool of choice). Focus on drawing the energy through you and direct it into your blade. Circle slowly from north, deosil, three times.

I cast this Circle once in the name of the Young Lord and the Maiden.
I cast this Circle twice in the name of the Father and the Mother.
I cast this Circle thrice in the name of the Sage and the Crone.

Turn to the North and say:

I invoke thee, Spirits of the Earth, you who are bone and stone and crystal, you who are rock and tree and branch and leaf. I invoke thee, you who are deepest caverns to the highest mountaintops. Come to me and bring with you your stability, your manifestation, your abundance and prosperity. Come to these rites, Spirits of Earth. Welcome and Blessed Be.

Turn to the East and say:

I invoke thee, Spirits of the Wind, you who are the chill breeze, you who are mist and fog and vapor and the gale of the hurricane. I invoke thee, you who are the rising winds and the gentle calm. Come to me and bring with you your keen insight and clarity of mind. Sweep through and remove stagnation and bring new beginnings. Come to these rites, Spirits of Wind. Welcome and Blessed Be.

Turn to the South and say:

I invoke thee, Spirits of Flame, you who are the crackling bonfire, you who are warmth of the hearth, the golden glow of the sun through the forest at midday. I invoke thee, you who are the glowing lava and the heat of the desert sands. Come to me and bring with you your passion and creativity, your healing and transformation. Come to these rites, Spirits of Flame. Welcome and Blessed Be.

Turn to the West and say:

I invoke thee, Spirits of the Water, you who are the raging river, you who are the crashing ocean breakers and the still pool of the grotto. I invoke thee, you who are the tears of our body, the rain kissing our brow. Come to me and bring with you joy and sorrow, laughter and tears, peace and enthusiasm. Lead me into the hidden depths of my psyche and guide the way into my heart. Come to these rites, Spirits of Water. Welcome and Blessed Be.

DEVOKING ELEMENTS AND OPENING THE CIRCLE

When the ritual is over, you will most likely want to devoke the Elements and open the Circle. This will open the energy pathways. At times I leave certain Circles intact, to settle into the walls of the house.

Turn to the West and say:

Spirits of the Water, Spirits of the Ocean, thank you for attending our Circle. Go if you must, stay if you will, hail and farewell.

Turn to the South and say:

Spirits of Flame, Spirits of the Fire, thank you for attending our Circle. Go if you must, stay if you will, hail and farewell.

Turn to the East and say:

Spirits of the Wind, Spirits of the Air, thank you for attending our Circle. Go if you must, stay if you will, hail and farewell.

Turn to the North and say:

Spirits of the Earth, Spirits of the Mountains, thank you for attending our Circle. Go if you must, stay if you will, hail and farewell.

Take your broom or use your hand, and slowly turn widdershins while envisioning the ring of energy opening. If you cast the Circle thrice, then devoke it with three turns; if you cast it once, then devoke it with one turn. Say:

This Circle is open but unbroken.
Merry Meet, Merry Part, and Merry Meet again!

SMUDGING

Smudging is using smoke to cleanse the energy/aura of things. You will want to use either a stick of incense, some granular incense on a piece of charcoal specifically designed for smudging, or a smudge stick (usually a bundle of sage, or sage and lavender, or sweet-grass). Make sure not to let the sparks fly onto clothing, and don't hold the smudge stick so close to someone's skin that you burn them—and be considerate enough to ask if people have allergies before you light up frankincense.

DRAWING-DOWN POSITION

Stand with your legs separated, feet firmly planted on the floor. Keep your back comfortably straight and your chin up, your gaze toward the ceiling. Your arms may be extended out to the side, palms up in a receiving position, or you may bend your elbows at your sides, with your palms open and facing the ceiling. The drawing–down position seems to be advantageous in opening the aura and body in order to receive energy from outside oneself.

MOON AND SUN WATER

Moon water is water that has been charged under the moon's energy. Sun water is water charged by the light of the sun.

FULL MOON WATER

Fill a glass jar with water. Add a moonstone to the jar and cap the jar. Three days before the Full Moon, set the jar outside at night where it can capture the moon's rays (it doesn't matter if the sky is overcast). Bring it in the following morning. Repeat this for the next two nights. After this, add water each month to the jar if needed and set the jar outside the night before the Full Moon to capture the moonlight.

NEW MOON WATER

Fill a glass jar with water. Add a piece of black onyx to the jar and cap the jar. Follow the directions for making Full Moon water, but set the jar outside during the New Moon (and the three days before it), instead of the Full Moon.

SUN WATER

Fill a glass jar with water. Add a piece of citrine or carnelian to the jar and cap the jar. Set it outside on three consecutive sunny days, taking it inside at dusk. For added strength, set the jar outside at dawn on the morning of the Summer Solstice. Use for solar rituals and spells.

---

1. *Embracing the Moon*, by Yasmine Galenorn, Llewellyn Worldwide, 1998.

References

SUGGESTED MUSIC FOR RITUALS AND MEDITATIONS

Dead Can Dance

Spiritchaser	Into the Labyrinth
Aion	The Serpent's Egg

Gabrielle Roth and The Mirrors

Tongues	Endless Wave
Totem	Initiation
Bones	Ritual
Waves	Luna
Zone Unknown	

Mike Oldfield

Tubular Bells

Phil Thornton and Hossam Ramsy

Eternal Egypt

Suvarna

Fire of the Oracle

SUGGESTED VIDEOTAPES

Aria; 1987: Ten vignettes based on operatic drama; erotica.

Bellydance! Magical Motion with Atéa; 1998: A good beginner's guide to bellydancing; easy to understand.

Kama Sutra: A Tale of Love; Director: Mira Nair; 1997 (Unrated): A spectacular love story set in sixteenth-century India. Incredible photography; brilliant settings; haunting eye candy; erotica.

Yoga for Round Bodies–Volumes 1 & 2; 1969: Yoga for larger bodies.

SUGGESTED READING

See the bibliography for reading recommendations.

ONLINE SITES—REFERENCE AND SHOPPING

Be aware that some online sites come and go like the wind; others stay around for years. If you do not find a site listed here, don't contact me about it, but perhaps try a search for the name under one of the search engines to see if it has moved to a new URL.

General Magick Sites and Magickal Shopping Sites
Circle Sanctuary: http://www.circlesanctuary.org/
Galenorn En/Visions: http://www.galenorn.com
Gothic Gardening: http://www.gothic.net/~malice/
JBL Statues: http://sacredsource.com/
A Mystical Grove: http://www.amysticalgrove.com/
New Moon Rising: http://www.celts.com/
    [*see also:* Magickal Magazines]
The Nine Houses of Gaia: http://www.9houses.org/
Pagans.org: http://www.pagans.org/
Ravens World: http://www.ravensworld.com
    [*see also:* Magickal Shopping Resources]

Sakti Dances: http://www.witch.drak.net/moonsoul/
Temple of Bastet: http://home.earthlink.net/~roscoecat/
The Wiccan-Pagan Times: http://www.twpt.com
Widdershins: http://www.widdershins.org/
    [*see also:* Magickal Magazines]
The Witches Voice: http://www.witchvox.com
Witch's Brew: http://www.witchs-brew.com/

BDSM Sites
Bedroom Bondage:
    http://www.bedroombondage.com/bedroom/index.htm
Different Loving: http://gloria-brame.com/diflove.htm
DungeonNet.com: http://www.dungeons.net/
Kinky Cards: http://www.kinkycards.com/
Meretrix Online: http://www.realm-of-shade.com/meretrix/
Seattle SM & Bondage Resources:
    http://www.halcyon.com/elf/seattle.html
The Wet Spot: http://www.wetspot.org/

Polyamory Sites
CAW (polyamory): http://www.caw.org/index.html
Loving More: http://lovemore.com/
The Polyamory Society: http://www.polyamorysociety.org/

Tantra and Sacred Sex Online Sites
The Church of Tantra: http://www.tantra.org/
The Goddess Temple: http://www.goddesstemple.com/
Sacred Sex: http://www.luckymojo.com/sacredsex.html
TantraWorks: http://www.tantraworks.com/tantrawk.html
Yoga Tantra Veda:
　　　http://www.geocities.com/athens/olympus/3588/yotaveda.html

Sex Shopping Sites
Adult Toy Chest: http://adulttoychest.com/
Good Vibrations: http://www.goodvibes.com/
　　　[1-800-289-8423 (1-800-BUY-VIBE)]
Lovers Package: http://www.loverspackage.com/
Toys In Babeland: http://www.babeland.com

Gay/Lesbian Resource Sites
Kurfew Club: http://www.kurfew.com/
PFLAG: http://www.pflag.org/
Ten Percent Bent: http://www.tenpercentbent.com/

Body Modification Sites
Body Modification Ezine: http://www.bme.freeq.com/
Body Play: http://www.bodyplay.com/bodyplay/
Ritual Magazine: http://www.ritualmag.co.uk/indexy.htm
Tattoo Rituals: http://www.metal-tiger.com/wu_tang_pca/tattoo.html

Dance Sites
The Art of Middle Eastern Dance: http://www.shira.net/
Chainmail & More: http://www.sblades.com/
Tribal Where?: http://tribalwhere.com/welcome.html

BBW Sites

BBW Magazine: http://www.bbwmagazine.com/
[P.O. Box 1297, Elk Grove, CA 95759]

Dimensions OnLine: http://www.pencomputing.com/dim/

Mode Magazine: http://www.modemag.com/
[P.O. Box 54275, Boulder, CO 80323-4275]

NAAFA: http://www.naafa.com
[P.O. Box 188620, Sacramento, CA 95818.
Phone: (916) 558-6880 Fax: (916) 558-6881]

Radiance Magazine: http://www.radiancemagazine.com
[P.O. Box 30246, Oakland, CA 94604.
Phone: (510) 482-0680, Fax: (510) 482-1576]

Activist Sites

ACLU: http://www.aclu.org

The Interfaith Alliance: http://www.tialliance.org/

The National Civil Rights Museum:
http://www.midsouth.rr.com/civilrights/

National Organization for Women: http://www.now.org/

Pagans Vote: http://www.pagansvote.org/

MAGICKAL SUPPLIES

Most of the shops listed here offer mail-order and/or online service and catalogs. Be aware, however, that retail shops go in and out of business with alarming frequency, and Web-based businesses seem even more prone to this on/off switch. Some of those listed may not be in service when you write to them. Others will spring up after this book has been published.

As far as local supplies go, look for candles in drugstores, stationery stores, grocery stores, and gift shops. Grocery stores and florists carry flowers, as do your friends' gardens. You can sometimes find essential oils in gift shops, perfume shops, etc., and crystals can be located in gift shops and rock shops. Gather your herbs wild or purchase them through grocery stores or food co-ops and herb shops, or go to local plant nurseries to get the plants themselves.

Unusual altar pieces can often be found at local import supply stores and secondhand stores. Altar cloths are easy: go to your favorite fabric shop and buy a piece of cloth large enough to cover your altar table.

Lastly, don't overlook the Yellow Pages. Look under metaphysical; herbs; books (bookstores often carry far more than books); lapidary supplies; and jewelry.

PAGAN/MAGICKAL STORES

Azure Green
48 Chester Rd.
Chester, MA 01011-9735

Eden Within
P.O. Box 667
Jamestown, NY 14702

Edge of the Circle Books
701 E. Pike
Seattle, WA 98122
(206) 726-1999

Gypsy Heaven
115 S. Main St.
New Hope, PA 18938
(catalog costs $3, refundable through
purchase; money orders only)

JBL Statues
http://sacredsource.com/
Phone: (800) 290-6203/
(804) 823-1515
Fax: (804) 823-7665

MoonScents & Magickal Blends
P.O. Box 3811588-LL
Cambridge, MA 02238

Raven's World
15600 NE 8th St.
Bellevue, WA 98008
(425) 644-7502

Sacred Source/JBL
Box WW
Crozet, VA 22932-0163
E-mail orders:
spirit@sacredsource.com

Serpentine Music Productions
P.O. Box 2564-L1
Sebastopol, CA 95473
(carries a wide variety of
hard-to-find Pagan music)

White Light Pentacles
P.O. Box 8163
Salem, MA 01971-8163

PAGAN/MAGICKAL JOURNALS AND MAGAZINES

The Beltane Papers
P.O. Box 29694
Bellingham, WA 98228-1694

Green Egg Magazine
212 So. Main St. #22-B
Willits, CA 95490
(707) 456-0332

New Moon Rising
http://www.celts.com/
P.O. Box 1731
Medford, OR 97501-0135
Phone: (541) 858-9404
Fax: (541) 779-8815

Open Ways
P.O. Box 14415
Portland, OR 97293-0415

The Sacred Horn
Unickorn Press
P.O. Box 143262
Anchorage, AK 99514-3262

SageWoman
P.O. Box 641LL
Point Arena, CA 95648

Shaman's Drum
P.O. Box 430
Willits, CA 95490-0430

Widdershins
http://www.widdershins.org/
Emerald City/Silver Moon
Productions
12345 Lake City Way NE, Suite 268
Seattle, WA 98125

Bibliography

Anderson, William, and Clive Hicks. *Green Man*. London/New York: HarperCollins, 1990.

Andrews, Ted. *Animal Speak*. St. Paul, MN: Llewellyn Worldwide, 1993.

Arons, Katie, and Jacqueline Shannon. *Sexy At Any Size*. New York: Fireside Books, 1999.

Conway, D.J. *The Ancient and Shining Ones*. St. Paul, MN: Llewellyn Worldwide, 1993.

———. *Lord of Light and Shadow*. St. Paul, MN: Llewellyn Worldwide, 1997.

Farrar, Janet, and Stewart Farrar. *The Witches' Goddess*. Custer, WA: Phoenix Publishing Inc., 1987.

———. *The Witches' God*. Custer, WA: Phoenix Publishing Inc., 1989.

Galenorn, Yasmine. "The Ceremony and Ritual Of Hula," *Llewellyn's 2000 Magickal Almanac*. St. Paul, MN: Llewellyn Worldwide, 1999.

———. *Dancing with the Sun*. St. Paul, MN: Llewellyn Worldwide, 1999.

———. *Embracing the Moon*. St. Paul, MN: Llewellyn Worldwide, 1998.

———. *Meditations on the Wheel of the Year*. Freedom, CA: The Crossing Press, 2002.

———. *Tarot Journeys*. St. Paul, MN: Llewellyn Worldwide, 1999.

Hirschmann, Jane, and Carol H. Munter. *When Women Stop Hating Their Bodies*. New York: Fawcett Columbine, 1995.

Hittleman, Richard. *Introduction to Yoga*. New York: Bantam, 1969.

Johnson, Carol. *Self-Esteem Comes in All Sizes*. New York: Doubleday, 1995.

MacLean, Helene. *Every Woman's Health*. New York: Doubleday Book & Music Clubs, 1980.

Meyer, Ken. *Real Women Don't Diet*. New York: Pinnacle Books, 1993.

Mifflin, Margot. *Bodies of Subversion*. New York: Juno Books, 1997.

Neel, Alexandra, and David Neel. *Magic and Mystery in Tibet*. New York: Dover Publications, 1971.

O'Brien, Paddy. *Yoga for Women*. San Francisco: Thorsons, 1994.

Tobias, Maxine, and John P. Sullivan. *Complete Stretching*. New York: Alfred A. Knopf, 1994.

Vale, V., and Andrea Juno. *Modern Primitives*. San Francisco: V/Search Publications, 1989.

MIND/BODY BOOKS BY THE CROSSING PRESS

200 Ways to Love the Body You Have

by Marcia Germaine Hutchinson

This companion to Marcia Hutchinson's bestselling *Transforming Body Image* consists of 200 pleasurable exercises from which you can choose at random. The new awareness these exercises bring will help you become focused and newly aware of your body as it is, and lead you to love the body you have.

$12.95 • Paper • ISBN 0-89594-999-7

All Women Are Healers: A Comprehensive Guide to Natural Healing

by Diane Stein

Stein's bestselling book on natural healing for women teaches women to take control of their bodies and lives and offers a wealth of information on various healing methods including Reiki, Reflexology, Polarity Balancing, and Homeopathy.

$14.95 • Paper • ISBN 0-89594-409-X

Inner Radiance, Outer Beauty

by Ambika Wauters

Ambika Wauters encourages women to seek and nurture themselves by dismissing unrealistic images of their bodies. She helps them find their archetype of beauty from within and express their inner awareness by transforming their physical appearance. Includes a 21–day program for regaining health and beauty.

$14.95 • Paper • ISBN 1-58091-080-7

Nature's Aphrodisiacs

by Nancy L. Nickell

Throughout the centuries, the search for Nature's aphrodisiacs has produced an array of substances guaranteed to heighten sexual desire and enhance performance—everything from oysters to powdered rhinoceros horn. Aphrodisiacs—what is fact, what is fiction? Are they based in science or on superstition? *Nature's Aphrodisiacs* examines these questions, separating fact from fiction, superstition from science.

$14.95 • Paper • ISBN 0-89594-890-7

MIND/BODY BOOKS BY THE CROSSING PRESS

Pocket Guide to Hatha Yoga
by Michele Picozzi

Hatha yoga is a holistic form of exercise tailor-made for modern Westerners. This guide offers a roadmap for the beginner and a comprehensive resource for the continuing yoga student.

$6.95 • Paper • ISBN 0-89594-911-3

Transforming Body Image: Learning to Love the Body You Have
by Marcia Hutchinson, Ed.D.

Uses step-by-step exercises for self-acceptance to integrate body, mind, and self-image. We recommend every woman read this book.
> —Ellen Bass and Laura Davis, authors of *The Courage to Heal*

$14.95 • Paper • ISBN 0-89594-172-4

SPIRITUALITY BOOKS BY THE CROSSING PRESS

Diane Stein's Guide to Goddess Craft
by Diane Stein

Originally published as *The Women's Spirituality Book*, this guide describes the beliefs and practices of the goddess craft as it relates to the daily lives of women. Designed to be useful to both men and women, it emphasizes achieving power and control through healing, visualization, Tarot, and the women's I Ching.

$12.95 • Paper • ISBN 1-58091-091-2

Essential Wicca
by Paul Tuitéan and Estelle Daniels

Focusing on earth, nature, and fertility, the religion embraces the values of learning, sexual equality, and divination. While most books on Wicca address either the solitary practitioner or those in covens, *Essential Wicca* covers all the bases—from core beliefs and practices, basic and group rituals, to festivals and gatherings, holy days, and rites of passage. A glossary with more than 200 entries and over 50 illustrations extends the meaning of the text.

$20.95 • Paper • ISBN 1-58091-099-8

Spirituality Books by The Crossing Press

The Heart of the Circle: A Guide to Drumming

by Holly Blue Hawkins

Holly Blue Hawkins will walk you through the process of finding a drum, taking care of it, calling a circle, setting an intention, and drumming together. She will also show you how to incorporate drumming into your spiritual practice. She offers you an invitation to explore rhythm in a free and spontaneous manner.

$12.95 • Paper • ISBN 1-58091-025-4

A Little Book of Altar Magic

by D. J. Conway

This third addition to the successful *A Little Book* series shows us how we, sometimes unknowingly, create altars in our daily surroundings. D. J. Conway offers information on the power and use of colors, and the historic and symbolic meaning of the elements, animals, and objects to help us create magical altars in our personal surroundings.

$9.95 • Paper • ISBN 1-58091-052-1

A Little Book of Love Magic

by Patricia Telesco

A cornucopia of lore, magic, and imaginative ritual designed to bring excitement and romance to your life. Patricia Telesco tells us how to use magic to manifest our hopes and dreams for romantic relationships, friendships, family relations, and passions for our work.

$9.95 • Paper • ISBN 0-89594-887-7

Wicca: The Complete Craft

by D. J. Conway

What is Wicca? D. J. Conway is the voice of reason who states clearly what the religion of Wicca is as well as what it is not. Whether already in the craft or just beginning, this book is the definitive resource for all those gentle souls looking for a guide to the Wiccan path.

$22.95 • Paper • ISBN 1-58091-092-0

To receive a current catalog from The Crossing Press,
call us toll-free at 1.800.777.1048
or visit our Web site at **www. crossingpress.com**

www.crossingpress.com

BROWSE through the Crossing Press Web site for information on upcoming titles, new releases, and backlist books including brief summaries, excerpts, author information, reviews, and more.

SHOP our store for all of our books and, coming soon, unusual, interesting, and hard-to-find sideline items related to Crossing's best-selling books!

READ informative articles by Crossing Press authors on all of our major topics of interest.

SIGN UP for our e-mail newsletter to receive late-breaking developments and special promotions from The Crossing Press.